W9-ABZ-257

Current Concepts of Somatization: Research and Clinical Perspectives

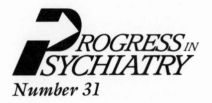

PROGRESS IN PSYCHIATRY

Number 31

David Spiegel, M.D.
Series Editor

Current Concepts of Somatization: Research and Clinical Perspectives

Edited by
Laurence J. Kirmayer, M.D., F.R.C.P.(C)
James M. Robbins, Ph.D.

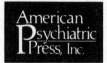

American Psychiatric Press, Inc.

Washington, DC
London, England

Note: The authors have worked to ensure that all information in this book concerning drug dosages, schedules, and routes of administration is accurate as of the time of publication and consistent with standards set by the U.S. Food and Drug Administration and the general medical community. As medical research and practice advance, however, therapeutic standards may change. For this reason and because human and mechanical errors sometimes occur, we recommend that readers follow the advice of a physician who is directly involved in their care or the care of a member of their family.

Copyright © 1991 American Psychiatric Press, Inc.
ALL RIGHTS RESERVED
Manufactured in the United States of America on acid-free paper.
First Printing
94 93 92 91 4 3 2 1

American Psychiatric Press, Inc.
1400 K Street, N.W., Washington, DC, 20005

Library of Congress Cataloging-in-Publication Data

Current concepts of somatization : research and clinical perspectives/edited by Laurence J. Kirmayer, James M. Robbins.
    p. cm.—(Progress in psychiatry: no. 31)
Includes bibliographical references and index.
ISBN 0-88048-198-6 (alk. paper)
1. Somatization disorder. I. Kirmayer, Laurence J., 1952– .
II. Robbins, James M., 1947– . III. Series.
    [DNLM: 1. Somatoform Disorders. WM 90 C9755]
RC552.S66C87 1991
616.85′2—dc20
DNLM/DLC
for Library of Congress   90-14492
                                                                    CIP
British Library Cataloguing in Publication Data

A CIP record is available from the British Library.

Contents

Contributors

Javier I. Escobar, M.D.
Professor and Associate Chairman (Research), Department of Psychiatry, University of Connecticut Health Center, Farmington, Connecticut

Horacio Fabrega, Jr., M.D.
Professor of Psychiatry and Anthropology, Department of Psychiatry, University of Pittsburgh School of Medicine, Western Psychiatric Institute and Clinic, Pittsburgh, Pennsylvania

Charles V. Ford, M.D.
Professor, Department of Psychiatry, School of Medicine, University of Alabama at Birmingham, Birmingham, Alabama

Robert Kellner, M.D., Ph.D., F.R.C. Psych.
Professor and Vice Chairman, Department of Psychiatry, University of New Mexico School of Medicine, Albuquerque, New Mexico

Laurence J. Kirmayer, M.D., F.R.C.P.(C)
Research Associate, Institute of Community and Family Psychiatry, Sir Mortimer B. Davis—Jewish General Hospital; Associate Professor, Department of Psychiatry, McGill University, Montreal, Quebec, Canada

Peter Manu, M.D.
Assistant Professor, Department of Internal Medicine, University of Connecticut Health Center, Farmington, Connecticut

Pamela E. Parker, M.D.
Assistant Professor, Department of Psychiatry, School of Medicine, University of Alabama at Birmingham, Birmingham, Alabama

James W. Pennebaker, Ph.D.
Professor, Department of Psychology, Southern Methodist University, Dallas, Texas

James M. Robbins, Ph.D.
Research Associate, Institute of Community and Family Psychiatry, Sir Mortimer B. Davis—Jewish General Hospital; Associate Professor, Departments of Psychiatry and Sociology, McGill University, Montreal, Quebec, Canada

Maritza Rubio-Stipec, M.A.
Assistant Professor, Department of Psychiatry, University of Puerto Rico, San Juan, Puerto Rico

Gregory E. Simon, M.D.
Assistant Investigator, Center for Health Studies, Group Health Cooperative of Puget Sound, Seattle, Washington

Marvin Swartz, M.D.
Associate Professor, Department of Psychiatry, Duke University, Durham, North Carolina

David Watson, Ph.D.
Associate Professor, Department of Psychology, Southern Methodist University, Dallas, Texas

Introduction to the Progress in Psychiatry Series

The Progress in Psychiatry Series is designed to capture in print the excitement that comes from assembling a diverse group of experts from various locations to examine in detail the newest information about a developing aspect of psychiatry. This series emerged as a collaboration between the American Psychiatric Association's (APA) Scientific Program Committee and the American Psychiatric Press, Inc. Great interest is generated by a number of the symposia presented each year at the APA annual meeting, and we realized that much of the information presented there, carefully assembled by people who are deeply immersed in a given area, would unfortunately not appear together in print. The symposia sessions at the annual meetings provide an unusual opportunity for experts who otherwise might not meet on the same platform to share their diverse viewpoints for a period of 3 hours. Some new themes are repeatedly reinforced and gain credence, while in other instances disagreements emerge, enabling the audience and now the reader to reach informed decisions about new directions in the field. The Progress in Psychiatry Series allows us to publish and capture some of the best of the symposia and thus provide an in-depth treatment of specific areas that might not otherwise be presented in broader review formats.

Psychiatry is by nature an interface discipline, combining the study of mind and brain, of individual and social environments, of the humane and the scientific. Therefore, progress in the field is rarely linear—it often comes from unexpected sources. Further, new developments emerge from an array of viewpoints that do not necessarily provide immediate agreement but rather expert examination of the issues. We intend to present innovative ideas and data that will enable you, the reader, to participate in this process.

We believe the Progress in Psychiatry Series will provide you with an opportunity to review timely new information in specific fields of interest as they are developing. We hope you find that the excitement of the presentations is captured in the written word and that this book proves to be informative and enjoyable reading.

David Spiegel, M.D.
Series Editor
Progress in Psychiatry Series

Progress in Psychiatry Series Titles

The Borderline: Current Empirical Research (#1)
Edited by Thomas H. McGlashan, M.D.

Premenstrual Syndrome: Current Findings and Future Directions (#2)
Edited by Howard J. Osofsky, M.D., Ph.D., and Susan J. Blumenthal, M.D.

Treatment of Affective Disorders in the Elderly (#3)
Edited by Charles A. Shamoian, M.D.

Post-Traumatic Stress Disorder in Children (#4)
Edited by Spencer Eth, M.D., and Robert S. Pynoos, M.D., M.P.H.

The Psychiatric Implications of Menstruation (#5)
Edited by Judith H. Gold, M.D., F.R.C.P. (C)

Can Schizophrenia Be Localized in the Brain? (#6)
Edited by Nancy C. Andreasen, M.D., Ph.D.

Medical Mimics of Psychiatric Disorders (#7)
Edited by Irl Extein, M.D., and Mark S. Gold, M.D.

Biopsychosocial Aspects of Bereavement (#8)
Edited by Sidney Zisook, M.D.

Psychiatric Pharmacosciences of Children and Adolescents (#9)
Edited by Charles Popper, M.D.

Psychobiology of Bulimia (#10)
Edited by James I. Hudson, M.D., and Harrison G. Pope, Jr., M.D.

Cerebral Hemisphere Function in Depression (#11)
Edited by Marcel Kinsbourne, M.D.

Eating Behavior in Eating Disorders (#12)
Edited by B. Timothy Walsh, M.D.

Tardive Dyskinesia: Biological Mechanisms and Clinical Aspects (#13)
Edited by Marion E. Wolf, M.D., and Aron D. Mosnaim, Ph.D.

Current Approaches to the Prediction of Violence (#14)
Edited by David A. Brizer, M.D., and Martha L. Crowner, M.D.

Treatment of Tricyclic-Resistant Depression (#15)
Edited by Irl L. Extein, M.D.

Depressive Disorders and Immunity (#16)
Edited by Andrew H. Miller, M.D.

Chapter 1

Introduction: Concepts of Somatization

Laurence J. Kirmayer, M.D., F.R.C.P.(C),
James M. Robbins, Ph.D.

S omatization is a term used to cover a broad range of common clinical situations: patients who present clinically with exclusively physical symptoms despite demonstrable psychosocial problems or emotional distress; patients who worry or are convinced that they are physically ill without evidence of disease; and people with a pattern of frequent unexplained or functional somatic symptoms that prompt help seeking and cause disability (Katon et al. 1982; Kellner 1990; Kirmayer 1984, 1986; Kleinman 1977; Lipowski 1968). The concept of somatization groups these different situations together on the assumption that what they have in common is that medically unexplained bodily distress is related to underlying psychiatric, psychological, or social problems.

Somatization in its various guises is an extremely common problem in all areas of medicine (Ford 1983; Kellner 1986; Lipowski 1988). It is also a major public health problem—functional symptoms are among the leading causes of work and social disability. Patients with recurrent unexplained somatic symptoms may be extensively investigated, be hospitalized, and undergo invasive diagnostic and surgical procedures and arduous medical treatments that are costly and can lead to serious iatrogenic disease. People with high levels of worry about being sick may use health care services inappropriately and may be more prone to suffer from the disabling effects of any disease they contract. Somatized depression and anxiety disorders are poorly recognized by primary care providers, leading to undertreatment with excess morbidity and chronicity.

Somatization may appear to be uncommon in specialized psychiatric clinics, where patients are referred or screened for their

Preparation of this chapter was aided by a grant from the Conseil québecois de la recherche sociale.

1

psychiatric symptomatology and "psychological mindedness." However, the impression of a low prevalence of somatization in this setting may be an artifact of psychiatric disinterest in somatic distress (Fabrega et al. 1988). The move of psychiatry back into general hospitals and the subsequent renaissance of consultation-liaison psychiatry, along with the recognition that the primary care system is essential to the delivery of mental health care, have made somatization a central problem for psychiatry and medicine.

In this volume we bring together current workers in this area to survey what has been accomplished, and outline the prospects for future research and advances in clinical practice.

FROM PSYCHOSOMATICS TO SOMATIZATION

Psychosomatic medicine has traditionally been concerned with investigating and treating the psychological determinants of disease. Psychodynamic theory attempted to study the role of specific psychological conflicts or personality dimensions in diseases. This strategy did not live up to its promise and had the unfortunate effect of encouraging clinicians to think of certain diseases as being especially "psychosomatic" in nature. Contemporary epidemiologic and psychophysiological research provides ample evidence of the non-specific effects of stress on the cause and course of disease. In fact, psychological and social effects on physiology are ubiquitous and have been found to play a potential role in virtually every disease studied. The recognition that there is no unique class of psychosomatic disorders—only particular clinical instances in which psychosocial factors play an overriding role in causing or aggravating a patient's condition—led to the elimination of the category of psychophysiological disorders from the *Diagnostic and Statistical Manual of Mental Disorders,* 3rd Edition (DSM-III) (American Psychiatric Association 1980) and the substitution of the label "psychological factors affecting physical condition." This term can be applied to clinical situations rather than to disease categories, encouraging physicians to think of psychosomatic process as a dimension of any disease.

Whereas psychosomatic theory is concerned with disease causation, somatization focuses attention on the experience and expression of illness. While earlier definitions of somatization simply assumed the psychosocial origins of functional somatic distress, this causal inference is, in fact, often difficult to verify both in research and in clinical practice. Lipowski (1988) has recently amended his original definition of somatization as "the tendency to experience, conceptualize, and/or communicate psychological states or contents as bodily sensations, functional changes, or somatic metaphors" (Lipowski 1968, p. 413) to make it more purely descriptive. Somatization is thus defined as "the tendency to experience and communicate somatic distress and symptoms unaccounted for by pathological findings, to attribute them to physical illness, and to seek medical help for them" (Lipowski 1988, p. 1359). As such, somatization is properly viewed as a variation in illness behavior and help seeking. The relationship of somatization to psychiatric disorder or psychosocial stress then becomes an empirical question rather than part of the definition.

SOMATIZATION AS SYMPTOM OR DISORDER

Psychodynamic theory confounded a mechanism of symptom production ("conversion"), a clinical presentation of multiple unexplained somatic symptoms in many different organ systems ("hysteria"), and a dramatic personality style with much amplification or exaggeration of distress ("hysterical personality") (Chodoff 1974; Slavney 1990). In the development of DSM-III, the classic concept of hysteria was "split asunder" to develop concepts of several distinct "somatoform" disorders—that is, problems claimed by psychiatry with predominantly somatic symptomatology (Hyler and Spitzer 1978). With the appearance of DMS-III-R (American Psychiatric Association 1987) these disorders underwent further revision to yield the current categories of conversion, somatization, body dysmorphic disorders, somatoform pain and undifferentiated somatoform disorders, somatoform disorder not otherwise specified, and hypochondriasis. The diagnostic validity and clinical utility of most of these categories remain to be established.

Conversion Disorder

Conversion symptoms are losses or alterations in bodily function that mimic physical disease, particularly neurological disorders such as blindness, deafness, anosmia, anesthesia, paralysis, ataxia, seizures, or loss of consciousness. The DSM-III diagnostic criteria included the requirement that the symptoms were caused by psychological conflict and/or had obvious symbolic significance. DSM-III also allowed that the psychological causation of conversion symptoms could be a result of the social benefits that accrued from the illness. Recognizing that psychological causation is difficult to verify and that secondary gain may be a feature of all illness, the architects of DSM-III-R simplified the judgment of psychological etiology, which now rests solely on the observation of a temporal relationship between salient psychosocial stressors and the onset or exacerbation of symptoms. Conversion is distinguished from factitious illness by the impression that the person does not consciously produce the symptom.

In actual practice the criterion of recent stressors does not discriminate conversion symptoms from those of other organic diseases that may be aggravated by stress. To distinguish conversion from organic disease the diagnostician must then fall back on a variety of system-specific maneuvers to rule out organic disease and to demonstrate that the pattern of symptomatology follows the patient's presumptive model of bodily functioning rather the established neurological pathways (Engel 1970).

As early as 1895, in the *Project for a Scientific Psychology*, Freud distinguished between somatic symptoms that were directly caused by excessive nervous activity without psychological mediation (the actual neuroses) and those that were indirectly caused by intrapsychic conflict (the neurosis of hysteria) (Sulloway 1979). The notion of the "transduction" of nervous activity into somatic disease is still common in psychosomatic theory. Some accounts of alexithymia, for example, imply that if strong emotions cannot be symbolically transformed and given verbal expression, they are "discharged" along autonomic pathways, causing physiological disorders (Nemiah 1977; Taylor 1984).

Freud applied the term "conversion" to the psychological mechanism whereby an accumulation of nervous energy, associated with unexpressed emotion, was repressed (pushed out of consciousness) and transformed into a somatic discharge creating bodily symptoms. Conversion differed from the direct somatic effects of the actual neuroses by involving psychological mediation. This distinction conferred on the somatic symptoms of conversion their symbolic meaning as communications or indices of underlying conflict.

Freud's early theories invoked quantities of psychic energy that have no simple physiological correlate in contemporary models of the brain. In place of energy metaphors, contemporary views of functional symptoms propose that cognitive processes of self-appraisal may lead to prolonged affective states of anxiety, effortful striving, or depression and demoralization (Lazarus and Folkman 1984). These affective states themselves are associated with specific patterns of physiological activation that may disrupt normal function by uncovering constitutional vulnerabilities or aggravating preexisting disease.

Similarly, current views of the production of conversion symptoms emphasize dissociative cognitive mechanisms similar to those evoked in hypnosis (Hilgard 1977). Conversion symptoms typically occur at times of great stress when spontaneous dissociation may be a method of coping. The form of conversion symptoms reflects patients' expectations and knowledge of disease (Raskin et al. 1966). The alteration of self-awareness that occurs in dissociation makes the symptom "ego-alien"—a "happening to" (the patient experiences the symptom as something that happens to him or her) rather than a voluntary act. In common with many stress-related symptoms, the majority of unilateral conversion symptoms affect the left side of the body in right-handed individuals, suggesting the mediation of the non-dominant cerebral hemisphere (Sackeim and Weber 1982).

Conversion symptoms are extremely common in the general population and in individuals with preexisting organic disease (Goodwin and Guze 1989; Watson and Buranen 1979a). Somatization disorder, histrionic personality disorder (Lilienfeld et al. 1986), high hypnotic susceptibility (Bliss 1984), and a history of other dissociative reactions (Watson and Tilleskjor 1983) are associated with conversion symptoms. The diagnosis of conversion is notoriously unreliable unless it is made in the context of a history of similar recurrent medically unexplained symptoms or somatization disorder (Raskin et al. 1966; Slater 1965; Watson and Buranen 1979b). Based, as it most often is, on a single acute episode, conversion is best thought of as a sporadic symptom with no specific psychopathological significance rather than as a discrete syndrome or disorder.

While the pseudoneurological symptoms of conversion disorder may reflect alterations in attention and somatomotor control, other functional somatic symptoms presumably involve different neurophysiological processes specific to the organ systems involved. Conversion symptoms and other functional somatic disorders thus may rise from mechanisms that are in themselves distinct from whatever unifying factor might account for the varied symptomatology of somatization disorder.

Somatization Disorder

The view of hysteria as a discrete syndrome of multiple somatic complaints has its modern origins in Briquet's *Traité clinique et thérapeutique de l'hystérie* (1859) (Mai and Merskey 1980). Owing largely to the vigorous research efforts of the Washington University research group in St. Louis (Guze 1967), the concept of Briquet's syndrome was incorporated into DSM-III as somatization disorder. This is described as a chronic disorder of multiple unexplained medical symptoms, starting before the age of 30, found primarily in women, and leading to persistent help seeking, medication use, disability, and iatrogenic disease. Common symptoms include musculoskeletal pains, gastrointestinal complaints, cardiopulmonary symptoms, pseudoneurological symptoms (e.g., numbness, paresthesia, loss of vision), menstrual problems, and sexual problems. Guze's original criteria for Briquet's syndrome required 20 medically unexplained symptoms in nine different groups (roughly sorted by functional system) (Perley and Guze 1962). The DSM-III definition of somatization disorder simplified this scheme by limiting the symptom list to the 37 items that best discriminated patients with Briquet's syndrome from those with other disorders. Possible confounding with depressive and anxiety disorders was reduced by eliminating some symptoms characteristic of these disorders. The number of symptoms required to reach criterion was reduced to 14 for women and 12 for men (the difference aimed to correct for any bias due to the inclusion of four symptoms unique to the female reproductive system). DSM-III-R (American Psychiatric Association 1987) has further simplified the criteria for somatization disorder, requiring 13 symptoms for either sex while retaining the female sex-specific items. Seven items are identified as an abbreviated screening measure: vomiting (other than during pregnancy), pain in extremities, short-ness of breath when not exerting, amnesia, difficulty swallowing, burning sensation in sexual organs or rectum (other than during intercourse), and painful menstruation. The presence of any two of these screening symptoms indicates a high likelihood that the full criteria for somatization disorder will be met (Smith and Brown 1990).

Despite the proposal of such abbreviated measures, it remains unclear what effect reducing the symptom level criterion from Briquet's syndrome to somatization disorder has had on the nature of the cases identified. Further, because of some nonoverlap in symptoms, it is possible to fulfill the criteria for Briquet's syndrome but not for DSM-III somatization disorder or vice versa. Cloninger et al. (1986) found that of 123 women who received diagnoses of either Briquet's syndrome or somatization disorder, 21% had somatization disorder only and 16% had Briquet's only. Familial aggregation of the disorder was found among patients with Briquet's syndrome but not among patients with somatization disorder. The inclusion of depressive and anxiety symptoms in the definition of Briquet's syndrome, along with the higher level of symptomatology required for diagnosis, tends to select a more homogeneous group of patients with a stronger familial predisposition toward a pattern of generalized somatic and emotional distress. Briquet's syndrome patients are likely to have histories of both major affective and anxiety disorders (Orenstein 1989). This may be because the inclusion of such symptoms as panic attacks, nervousness, fears, depressed feelings, crying easily, hopelessness, and thoughts about death or suicide in the criteria for Briquet's syndrome makes it a stronger index of negative affectivity—a heritable trait related to somatization, anxiety, and depression (cf. Pennebaker and Watson, Chapter 2, this volume). The reduction of the criterion level below that of DSM-III-R—as in the "subsyndromal somatization disorder" proposed by Escobar et al. (1989)—probably defines a much more heterogeneous population that includes individuals with discrete functional somatic syndromes and somatic symptoms secondary to an affective or anxiety disorder (cf. Kirmayer and Robbins, Chapter 5, this volume).

Body Dysmorphic Disorder

Called "dysmorphophobia" in the past, DSM-III-R defines this disorder as a preoccupation with some imagined defect in appearance in a normal-appearing person. If the belief is of delusional proportions, then it is separately classified as *delusional disorder, somatic type*. In practice, this distinction is difficult to make (de Leon et al. 1989). The alterations in body image that accompany anorexia nervosa or transsexualism are explicitly excluded. Monosymptomatic hypochondriacal psychosis is a related but more heterogeneous category comprising patients with delusions of an offensive body odor, nonexistent anatomical abnormalities, or an infestation with insects or parasites (Munro 1988). Clearly, dysmorphophobia is a symptom not a syndrome; when mild, it usually reflects social anxiety and broader deficits in self-esteem. When severe, dysmorphophobia is often a feature of a psychotic disorder—schizophrenia, major depression, paranoid disorder, or an organic brain syndrome.

Somatoform Pain Disorder

The DSM-III criteria for psychogenic pain disorder paralleled those for conversion disorder. With increasing recognition of the difficulty in distinguishing "psychogenic" from pathogenic pain, the criterion of a psychological cause has been dropped. Instead, DSM-III-R merely requires that the patient have been preoccupied with pain for at least 6 months and that there be no organic pathology or pathophysiological mechanism to account for the pain, or, when there is organic pathology, that the degree of pain or disability is "grossly in excess of what would be expected from the physical findings" (American Psychiatric Association 1987, p. 266). These criteria remain problematic, because the judgment of whether a pain syndrome can be physiologically explained is largely a function of current diagnostic fashion and popular theories. For example, DSM-III-R states that the pain of muscle contraction headache is not to be counted as somatoform pain disorder because a mechanism is known (indeed, is stipulated in the name). In reality, many cases of "idiopathic" musculoskeletal pains can be plausibly attributed to muscle tension with little possibility of objective clinical verification. Further, there is a low correlation between extent of tissue injury and pain, and, consequently, clinicians' ability to judge appropriate levels of pain in organic disease is poor. While organic contributors can be found for many patients with chronic pain, psychological factors always play a prominent role in the intensity and quality of pain experience (Melzack and Wall 1982).

Building on the proposal of Engel (1959), Blumer and Heilbronn (1982) described a "pain-prone disorder" characterized by hypochondriacal worry, denial of psychological conflicts, idealization of self and family, "workaholism," and a high frequency of major depressive disorder. Other research has reported a high prevalence of alexithymic traits in chronic pain patients, that is, a lack of recollection of dreams and fantasy, and difficulty with symbolic expressions of emotion and conflict resolution (Catchlove et al. 1985). However, chronic-pain patients comprise a very heterogeneous population (Williams and Spitzer 1982). Chronic pain may be a manifestation of an underlying major depression in a small proportion of patients. Far more commonly, depression results from persistent pain, which it then exacerbates. Treatment of concomitant depression then reduces but does not eliminate chronic pain. Premorbid differences in personality may influence individuals' ability to cope with persistent pain, but the bodily preoccupation of chronic-pain patients, along with many apparent similarities in personality, likely reflects the way in which unrelenting pain comes to dominate consciousness and alter the self concept.

Hypochondriasis

In DSM-III-R, hypochondriasis is defined as a "preoccupation with the fear of having, or the belief that one has, a serious disease, based on the person's interpretation of physical signs or sensations as evidence of physical illness" (American Psychiatric Association 1987, p. 259). This fear or belief occurs in the absence of a physical disorder that could account for the patient's concerns and persists despite medical reassurance.

Measures of hypochondriasis tend to include dimensions of worry about getting ill, conviction of having a disease, self-perception of being sensitive to sensations, and preoccupation with bodily symptoms (Barsky et al. 1986; Pilowsky 1967; Pilowsky and Spence 1983). Hypochondriacal behavior has been attributed to an amplifying bodily style that leads to increased symptom experience, symptom reporting, and help seeking (Barsky and Klerman 1983). However, hypochondriasis is often associated with other anxiety or depressive disorders, and some authorities have argued that it should be viewed as a symptom secondary to these disorders rather than an entity in its own right (Kenyon 1976).

Hypochondriasis can be an acute and transient symptom or an enduring stance toward one's body and health (Barsky et al. 1990). When bodily distress is felt to be due to a serious illness, hypochondriacal worry can be intense and even disabling, yet can quickly respond to medical investigation and reassurance. In some individuals hypochondriasis may be associated with enduring personality traits that leave the person with a constant sense of physical vulnerability and fear of illness. In these cases hypochondriasis could be viewed as a symptom of an underlying personality disorder.

Undifferentiated Somatoform Disorder

This category was created for patients with one or more physical complaints that are either medically unexplained or from which these patients suffer disability or help seeking that is "grossly in excess of what would be expected from the physical findings" (American Psychiatric Association 1987, p. 266). This category would include the abridged somatization disorder defined by Escobar et al. (1989; Chapter 4, this volume). Although defined as a residual category, the vast majority of patients with persistent somatization fall into this category.

Conclusion

With the possible exception of somatization disorder per se, the somatoform disorders appear to be best thought of as symptoms or patterns of reaction rather than discrete disorders with an intrinsic natural history. This suggests that we might shift our attention from efforts to characterize disorders to an attempt to better understand the underlying pathological processes that may result in functional somatic distress.

SOMATIZATION AS ILLNESS BEHAVIOR

As noted above, somatization can be viewed as a pattern of illness behavior. The term *illness behavior* was introduced by the medical sociologist David Mechanic to refer to "the ways in which given symptoms may be differently perceived, evaluated and acted (or not acted) upon by different kinds of persons" (Mechanic 1962, p. 189). This definition includes cognitive or intrapsychic processes as well as overt behaviors. The illness behavior perspective directs attention to observed patterns of response to bodily sensations and somatic distress. Variations among individuals in their overt behavior in response to illness can then presumably be understood in terms of psychological and social processes.

Pilowsky (1969, 1990) extended the illness-behavior concept to problematic clinical situations, calling somatization, exaggeration, or denial of illness "abnormal illness behavior." He has developed a typology of clinical problems that are deviations in illness behavior (Pilowsky 1978). However, there are a number of problems with this proposal (Mayou 1989). Illness behavior, as the term was introduced, is a nonnormative, descriptive concept. There are few established norms to justify the judgment that a patient's thoughts and actions are abnormal. Labeling patients' behavior "abnormal" shifts attention away from those social contextual factors—such as doctor-patient interaction or the exigencies of the health care and insurance/compensation systems—that may account for individual differences.

There is a further methodological problem with the term "abnormal illness behavior." Pilowsky and others (1979, 1983; Kellner 1987) have developed self-report and interviewer-rated questionnaires for illness behavior. These questionnaires usually sample only a limited range of patients' symptoms, mood, and attitudes and very little of their actual behavior (e.g., pattern of help seeking or way of coping). As such, the scales that have been generated are measures of health status or attitudes rather than of illness behavior per se. In the absence of additional information about patients' past history, current physical condition, and social context, it is rarely possible to characterize illness behavior from these measures. For example, hypochondriasis scales in fact largely measure illness worry. Only when disease that could reasonably account for the patient's worry has been ruled out, is it warranted to apply the term hypochondriasis (Costa and McCrae 1985; Zonderman et al. 1985). A scale that does attempt to address behavioral or communicative aspects of the response to illness, the Illness Behavior Inventory, has been developed by Turkat and Pettigrew (1983).

Despite efforts to define somatoform disorders in nonnormative terms, concepts of somatization retain a normative dimension. Hypochondriasis is illness worry that is judged to be disproportionate to the patient's objective disease. It thus reflects societal standards of stoicism, minimization or "normalization," and denial. The concept of somatization as a style of symptom presentation reflects normative standards for the attribution and explanation of distress. People in conflict are expected to relate their symptoms to that conflict—notwithstanding the fact that a marital argument may be quickly overshadowed by the headache it provokes. When patients with obvious psychosocial problems insist that their somatic symptoms are the "real," primary, or "only" problem, they may be viewed as somatizing. Even functional symptoms are those for which contemporary medicine has no widely accepted organic explanation, and the validity of marginal diagnostic categories—such as chronic fatigue syndrome or total allergy syndrome—reflects normative conventions in the medical and scientific communities. Thus, the clinical judgment that a patient is somatizing is open to a wide range of extraneous social factors including physician and institutional biases that are independent of the patient's pattern of illness behavior (Kirmayer 1987, 1988).

Ultimately, the view of somatization as illness behavior leads outward toward interpersonal processes and larger social structural factors. Medical anthropologists have made clear the ways in which bodily idioms of distress serve as a symbolic means of both social regulation and protest or contestation (Kleinman 1977, 1986; Scheper-Hughes and Lock 1987). While clinicians are, of necessity, concerned first with the patient before them, accurate diagnosis and effective treatment may require attention to the wider social context that can engender and sustain medically inexplicable somatic distress.

FORMS OF SOMATIZATION

What DSM-III split asunder, the broad concept of somatization puts back together. Is it better to lump or to split the somatoform disorders? In favor of lumping, there may be important commonalities between syndromes: similar psychological processes may be at work, and the clinical and social significance of medically unexplained physical symptoms, hypochondriacal worry, and somatized depression or anxiety may be similar. However, these putative similarities are research questions that can be addressed only by comparative studies of homogeneous groups (or by studies that adequately control for confounding factors). This is the spirit in which current psychiatric nosology has attempted to define research diagnostic criteria.

We examined the co-occurrence of three forms of somatization in a sample of 700 family-medicine patients (Kirmayer and Robbins, in press). Somatization was defined as 1) *functional somatization* (i.e., a history of high levels of medically unexplained somatic symptomatology on the National Institute of Mental Health [NIMH] Diagnostic Interview Schedule [DIS; Robins et al. 1981], using the abridged somatization criteria proposed by Escobar et al. [1989]); 2) *hypochondriacal somatization* (i.e., high levels of worry about having a serious illness in the absence of evidence for a serious illness [hypochondriasis]); and 3) *presenting somatization* (i.e., exclusively somatic clinical presentations in patients with evidence of a current major depression or anxiety disorder on the DIS).

One-fourth of the patients attending a family medicine clinic on a self-initiated visit met criteria for one or more forms of somatization. Although there was substantial overlap between forms of somatization, the majority of patients met criteria for only one form of somatization. Furthermore, the types of patients in each category were different: functional somatizers were more frequently women, while there was no preponderance of women in either hypochondriacal or presenting somatizers. Functional somatizers and hypochondriacal somatizers reported high levels of somatic symptomatology on the Symptom Checklist-90 (SCL-90; Derogatis et al. 1974) but presenting somatizers did not. As might be expected from the definition, presenting somatizers reported elevated levels of depressive symptomatology on the Center for Epidemiologic Studies Depression (CES-D) scale (Roberts and Vernon 1983) (although not nearly as high as depressed patients who presented with psychosocial complaints), but hypochondriacal patients reported levels of depression just as high without fulfilling DIS criteria for a depressive disorder.

The picture that emerges from this study is of three distinct forms of somatization reflecting different pathological processes. A history of functional symptoms, while it is associated with a continuing tendency to present medically inexplicable symptomatology, is not necessarily associated with either hypochondriasis or a current major depression or anxiety disorder. Hypochondriacal worry is associated with anxious or dysphoric mood but not exclusively with major depression or anxiety. Patients with somatic presentations of mood and anxiety disorders are most often neither chronic functional somatizers nor hypochondriacal individuals.

These forms of somatization may be related—an amplifying somatic style, for example, may aggravate functional somatic symptoms and lead to increased disability and health care utilization. A current major depression may increase somatic (vegetative) symptoms and give rise to hypochondriacal worry. Further, some of the nonoverlap between the three forms of somatization may reflect a temporal discrepancy—functional somatizers were not currently depressed or hypochondriacal but may be more likely to have been so in the past and to be so on a future occasion.

Although pure types are more common than mixed types of somatization, they may be less problematic for the clinician and harder to detect. The clinician's image of the prototypical somatizing patient may be based on those patients who suffer from all three forms described here, where the several processes may amplify each other to give rise to higher levels of distress and an intractable situation. Nevertheless, for research and clinical practice to advance, these conceptually distinct forms of somatization must be distinguished. That is what we have asked the contributors of this volume to do.

OUTLINE OF THIS VOLUME

James Pennebaker and David Watson, in Chapter 2, outline basic research in experimental psychology on the perception, interpretation, and reporting of somatic symptoms. These studies are just as relevant to patients coping with organic disease as to patients with problems of somatization. The authors provide the normative basis for understanding pathological extremes. In addition to discussing cognitive factors involving selective attention to bodily or environmental stimuli, they summarize evidence for individual differences in the tendency to experience dysphoric mood and somatic distress that may be linked to heritable traits and help explain gender differences in symptom experience and reporting. Drs. Pennebaker and Watson conclude with a discussion of the classification of somatoform disorders in DSM-III-R and methodological issues for future research.

In a wide-ranging overview (Chapter 3), Gregory Simon outlines four models of the relationship between psychiatric disorders, somatic distress, and health care utilization. He considers somatization as a psychological defense, the nonspecific amplification of distress, the tendency to seek care for common symptoms, and a consequence of the impact of the health care system itself. He then addresses the methodological problems of studying psychiatric comorbidity in somatizing patients. In a concluding section Dr. Simon maps out some of the therapeutic implications of alternative models of somatization and offers thoughtful guidelines for clinicians.

Javier Escobar and colleagues review recent epidemiologic work on the community prevalence and consequences of medically unexplained somatic symptoms in Chapter 4. They summarize results from the NIMH Epidemiologic Catchment Area studies and from a parallel survey in Puerto Rico on the psychiatric comorbidity, disability, and health care utilization associated with unexplained symptoms. They present the rationale for their proposal of an abridged somatization construct that may represent a *form fruste* (or "subsyndromal" version) of somatization disorder. A brief measure of medically unexplained symptoms that is being developed by the authors may serve as an unobtrusive screening tool for psychiatric distress in medical clinic populations of patients who may be more comfortable describing somatic symptoms than responding to direct inquiries about emotional distress.

In Chapter 5, we review recent work on the common functional somatic syndromes of fibromyalgia, irritable bowel, and chronic fatigue. Psychiatric morbidity is often found in clinical studies of these syndromes, but this may in part be because it leads to increased help seeking among people with milder forms of functional distress. Latent variable models offer a new way of studying relationships among superficially different syndromes. Preliminary results provide evidence for both discrete functional syndromes and important interrelationships with syndromes of somatic depression and anxiety.

In Chapter 6, we present further results based on a longitudinal study of 700 family-medicine patients. We provide evidence for distinct cognitive and social factors in three forms of somatization: functional symptoms, hypochondriacal worry, and somatic clinical presentations of mood or anxiety disorders. Of the three, functional somatization is most closely associated with subsequent health care utilization; hypochondriacal worry is most consistent with a negative, pessimistic self-image; and somatic presentations of psychiatric disorders are most likely to be found among patients without a psychosomatic cognitive schema that connects somatic and intrapsychic distress. These studies open the way to exploring the interaction among different forms of somatization.

Charles Ford and Pamela Parker, in Chapter 7, sketch the evolution of consultation-liaison psychiatry. They examine the place of somatoform disorders in general hospital psychiatry and outline current approaches to somatizing patients, including the development of specialized "med-psych" inpatient units and behavioral-medicine clinics as well as some specific modalities found helpful in these settings.

In Chapter 8, Robert Kellner reviews controlled trials of pharmacological and psychological treatments for patients with functional symptoms and hypochondriasis. Cognitive-educational approaches show promise in reducing the symptoms and disability associated with somatization. Contrary to the therapeutic nihilism that prevails in some quarters, Dr. Kellner's reading of the evidence suggests that somatizing patients are eminently treatable with appropriate psychotherapeutic methods.

In the penultimate chapter, Horacio Fabrega, Jr., critically explores the underlying cultural assumptions in our concepts of somatization. Arguing that the concept could only arise in a fundamentally dualistic medical system, he illustrates alternative views of the nature of illness in the great traditions of Ayurvedic, Chinese, and ancient Greek medicine. The challenge implicit in current work on somatization, then, is how to develop a truly comprehensive and nondualistic approach to medical care.

In the final chapter we take up the prospects for future research and advances in clinical practice. Promising research directions can be drawn from work in cognitive and social psychology, family interactional theory, and cross-cultural studies of idioms of distress. Psychological and social science research findings offer clinicians new ways to understand and treat somatization. In parallel with the development of technical interventions for symptom reduction and control, medicine has a broader therapeutic mandate: to allow patient and clinician together to make sense of suffering through the collaborative construction of personally and culturally coherent illness meanings (Kleinman 1988). The clinician who works with problems of somatization must master many languages to listen to the meanings of distress in personal, family, social, and cultural contexts.

REFERENCES

American Psychiatric Association: Diagnostic and Statistical Manual of Mental Disorders, 3rd Edition. Washington DC, American Psychiatric Association, 1980

American Psychiatric Association: Diagnostic and Statistical Manual of Mental Disorders, 3rd Edition, Revised. Washington DC, American Psychiatric Association, 1987

Barsky AJ, Klerman GL: Overview: hypochondriasis, bodily complaints, and somatic styles. Am J Psychiatry 140:273–283, 1983

Barsky AJ, Wyshak G, Klerman GL: Hypochondriasis: an evaluation of the DSM-III criteria in medical outpatients. Arch Gen Psychiatry 43:493–500, 1986

Barsky AJ, Wyshak G, Klerman GL: Transient hypochondriasis. Arch Gen Psychiatry 47:746–753, 1990

Bliss EL: Hysteria and hypnosis. J Nerv Ment Dis 172:203–206, 1984

Blumer D, Heilbronn M: Chronic pain as a variant of depressive disease. J Nerv Ment Dis 170:381–406, 1982

Catchlove RFH, Cohen KR, Braha RED, et al: Incidence and implications of alexithymia in chronic pain patients. J Nerv Ment Dis 173:246–248, 1985

Chodoff P: The diagnosis of hysteria: an overview. Am J Psychiatry 131:1073–1078, 1974

Cloninger CR, Martin RL, Guze SB, et al: A prospective follow-up study and family study of somatization in men and women. Am J Psychiatry 143:873–878, 1986

Costa PT Jr, McCrae RR: Hypochondriasis, neuroticism, and aging: when are somatic complaints unfounded? Am Psychol 40:19–28, 1985

de Leon J, Bott A, Simpson GM: Dysmorphophobia: body dysmorphic disorder or delusional disorder, somatic subtype? Compr Psychiatry 30:457–472, 1989

Derogatis LR, Lipman RS, Rickels K, et al: The Hopkins Symptom Checklist (HSCL): a self-report inventory. Behav Sci 19:1–15, 1974

Engel GL: Psychogenic pain and the pain-prone patient. Am J Med 26:899–918, 1959

Engel GL: Conversion symptoms, in Signs and Symptoms: Applied Pathologic Physiology and Clinical Interpretation, 5th Edition. Edited by MacBryde CM, Blacklow RS. Philadelphia, PA, JB Lippincott, 1970, pp 650–668

Escobar JI, Rubio-Stipec M, Canino G, et al: Somatic Symptom Index (SSI): a new and abridged somatization construct: prevalence and epidemiological correlates in two large community samples. J Nerv Ment Dis 177:140–146, 1989

Fabrega H Jr, Mezzich JE, Jacob R, et al: Somatoform disorder in a psychiatric setting. J Nerv Ment Dis 176:431–439, 1988

Ford CV: The Somatizing Disorders. New York, Elsevier, 1983

Goodwin DW, Guze SB: Psychiatric Diagnosis, 4th Edition. New York, Oxford University Press, 1989

Guze SB: The diagnosis of hysteria: what are we trying to do? Am J Psychiatry 124:491–498, 1967

Hilgard ER: Divided Consciousness: Multiple Controls in Human Thought and Action. New York, John Wiley, 1977

Hyler SE, Spitzer RL: Hysteria split asunder. Am J Psychiatry 135:1500–1504, 1978

Katon W, Kleinman A, Rosen G: Depression and somatization: a review. Am J Med 72:127–135, 241–247, 1982

Kellner R: Somatization and Hypochondriasis. New York, Praeger-Greenwood, 1986

Kellner R: Psychological measurements in somatization and abnormal illness behavior. Adv Psychosom Med 17:101–118, 1987

Kellner R: Somatization: theories and research. J Nerv Ment Dis 178:150–160, 1990

Kenyon F: Hypochondriacal states. Br J Psychiatry 129:1–14, 1976

Kirmayer LJ: Culture, affect and somatization. Transcultural Psychiatric Research Review 21:159–188, 237–262, 1984

Kirmayer LJ: Somatization and the social construction of illness experience, in Illness Behavior: A Multidisciplinary Model. Edited by McHugh S, Vallis TM. New York, Plenum, 1986, pp 111–133

Kirmayer LJ: Languages of suffering and healing: alexithymia as a social and cultural process. Transcultural Psychiatric Research Review 24:119–136, 1987

Kirmayer LJ: Mind and body as metaphors: hidden values in biomedicine, in Biomedicine Examined. Edited by Lock M, Gordon D. Dordrecht, The Netherlands, Kluwer, 1988, pp 57–92

Kirmayer LJ, Robbins JM: Three forms of somatization in primary care: prevalence, co-occurrence, and sociodemographic characteristics. J Nerv Ment Dis (in press)

Kleinman A: Depression, somatization and the "new cross-cultural psychiatry." Soc Sci Med 11:3–10, 1977

Kleinman A: Social Origins of Distress and Disease. New Haven, CT, Yale University Press, 1986

Kleinman A: The Illness Narratives: Suffering, Healing and the Human Condition. New York, Harper & Row, 1988

Lazarus R, Folkman S: Stress, Appraisal and Coping. New York, Springer, 1984

Lilienfeld SO, Van Valkenburg C, Larntz K, et al: The relationship of histrionic personality disorder to antisocial personality and somatization disorder. Am J Psychiatry 143:718–722, 1986

Lipowski ZJ: Review of consultation-liaison psychiatry and psychosomatic medicine, III: theoretical issues. Psychosom Med 30:395–422, 1968

Lipowski ZJ: Somatization: the concept and its clinical application. Am J Psychiatry 145:1358–1368, 1988

Lipowski ZJ: Somatization and depression. Psychosomatics 31:13–21, 1990

Mai FM, Merskey H: Briquet's Treatise on Hysteria: a synopsis and commentary. Arch Gen Psychiatry 37:1401–1404, 1980

Mayou R: Illness behavior and psychiatry. Gen Hosp Psychiatry 11:307–312, 1989

Mechanic D: The concept of illness behavior. J Chronic Dis 15:189–194, 1962

Melzack R, Wall P: The Challenge of Pain. Harmondsworth, Middlesex, Penguin Books, 1982

Munro A: Monosymptomatic hypochondriacal psychosis. Br J Psychiatry 153 (suppl 2): 37–40, 1988

Nemiah JC: Alexithymia: theoretical considerations. Psychother Psychosom 28:199–206, 1977

Orenstein H: Briquet's syndrome in association with depression and panic: a reconceptualization of Briquet's syndrome. Am J Psychiatry 146:334–338, 1989

Perley MJ, Guze SB: Hysteria—the stability and usefulness of clinical criteria. N Engl J Med 266:421–426, 1962

Pilowsky I: Dimensions of hypochondriasis. Br J Psychiatry 113:89–93, 1967

Pilowsky I: Abnormal illness behavior. Br J Med Psychol 42:347–351, 1969

Pilowsky I: A general classification of abnormal illness behaviours. Br J Med Psychol 51:131–137, 1978

Pilowsky I: The concept of abnormal illness behavior. Psychosomatics 31:207–213, 1990

Pilowsky I, Spence D: Manual for the Illness Behaviour Questionnaire, 2nd Edition. Adelaide, Australia, University of Adelaide, 1983

Pilowsky I, Murrell GC, Gordon A: The development of a screening method for abnormal illness behaviour. J Psychosom Res 23:203–207, 1979

Pilowsky I, Bassett D, Barrett R, et al: The illness behavior assessment schedule: reliability and validity. Int J Psychiatry Med 13:11–28, 1983

Raskin M, Talbott JA, Meyerson AT: Diagnosis of conversion reactions: predictive value of psychiatric criteria. JAMA 197:102–106, 1966

Roberts RE, Vernon SW: The Center for Epidemiologic Studies Depression scale: its use in a community sample. Am J Psychiatry 140:41–46, 1983

Robins LN, Helzer JE, Croughan J, et al: National Institute of Mental Health Diagnostic Interview Schedule: its history, characteristics, and validity. Arch Gen Psychiatry 38:381–389, 1981

Sackeim HA, Weber SL: Functional brain asymmetry in the regulation of emotion, in Handbook of Stress. Edited by Goldberger L, Breznitz S. New York, Free Press, 1982, pp 182–199

Scheper-Hughes N, Lock M: The mindful body: a prolegomenon to future work in medical anthropology. Med Anthropol 1:6–41, 1987

Slater E: Diagnosis of hysteria. Br Med J 1:1395–1399, 1965

Slavney PR: Perspectives on Hysteria. Baltimore, MD, Johns Hopkins University Press, 1990

Smith GR, Brown FW: Screening indexes in DSM-III-R somatization disorder. Gen Hosp Psychiatry 12:148–152, 1990

Sulloway F: Freud: Biologist of the Mind. New York, Basic Books, 1979

Taylor G: Alexithymia: concept, measurement, and implications for treatment. Am J Psychiatry 141:725–732, 1984

Turkat ID, Pettigrew IS: Development and validation of the Illness Behavior Inventory. Journal of Behavioral Assessment 5:35–47, 1983

Watson CG, Buranen C: The frequencies of conversion reaction symptoms. J Abnorm Psychol 88:209–211, 1979a

Watson CG, Buranen C: The frequency and identification of false positive conversion reactions. J Nerv Ment Dis 167:243–247, 1979b

Watson CG, Tilleskjor C: Interrelationships of conversion, psychogenic pain, and dissociative-disorder symptoms. J Consult Clin Psychol 51:788–789, 1983

Williams JBW, Spitzer RL: Idiopathic pain disorder: a critique of pain-prone disorder and a proposal for a revision of the DSM-III category psychogenic pain disorder. J Nerv Ment Dis 170:410–419, 1982

Zonderman AB, Heft MW, Costa PT Jr: Does the Illness Behavior Questionnaire measure abnormal illness behavior? Health Psychol 4:425–436, 1985

Chapter 2

The Psychology of Somatic Symptoms

James W. Pennebaker, Ph.D., David Watson, Ph.D.

The somatoform disorders are characterized by the awareness and reporting of physical symptoms. The underlying clinical assumption regarding most patients with somatization problems is that these individuals report a variety of physical complaints that lack a clear physiological basis. If these symptoms do not have clear physiological correlates, how do they arise? Whereas much of the research in this area has been devoted to creating a comprehensive taxonomy of the somatoform disorders in clinical samples, our strategy has been to understand the social and psychological bases of symptom reporting among relatively healthy individuals both in the laboratory and in naturalistic environments.

This chapter is divided into two parts. First, we review various psychological processes that influence the awareness and reporting of bodily sensations. Drawing on our own and others' work, we discuss the perceptual, dispositional, and genetic bases of symptom reporting. The remainder of the chapter is devoted to applying this knowledge of symptom reporting to future research projects focusing on somatoform disorders.

PERCEPTUAL, DISPOSITIONAL, AND GENETIC BASES OF SYMPTOM REPORTS

Although somatizing patients report a variety of symptoms that do not have a clear biological basis, the prevailing opinion is that their reports are subjectively real (Lipowski 1988; Robbins and Kirmayer 1986). That is, when individuals report symptoms and sensations, they subjectively experience significant bodily activity. The question that immediately comes to mind, then, concerns the perceptual information that influences how individuals attend to and interpret their body's ambiguous signals. Research that has addressed this issue has evolved considerably over the last century.

Preparation of this manuscript was aided by a grant from the National Science Foundation (BNS-8606764).

21

Symptom Reporting as a Perceptual Process

The laboratories of Wilhelm Wundt and Gustav Fechner yielded the first scientific investigations relevant to symptom perception. In developing the science of psychophysics, Wundt and others demonstrated a one-to-one correspondence between external stimuli and the perception of stimuli (Boring 1950). That is, when all extraneous variables were held constant, perceptions of light, sound, touch, and other sensory dimensions were mathematically related to the sources of the percepts.

J. J. Gibson (1979) was one of the first researchers to question the psychophysics tradition within perceptual psychology. The crux of his argument was that organisms rely on information from a variety of sources in order to perceive even the simplest stimulus arrays. Further, organisms are not passive recipients of information. Rather, they actively search the environment in order to understand it better and, consequently, to behave appropriately and efficiently.

Consider, for example, how individuals perceive the brightness of the moon at night. Of course, they rely heavily on their eyes and their visual systems in general. But the perception of the brightness of an object depends on much more than the stimulation of a portion of rods and cones within the retina. Visually, perception of brightness will also vary depending on the background of the sky, other visible objects, and the degree of adaptation to darkness. Beyond the visual system, the perception of brightness will also be affected by our beliefs about or needs concerning the object. For example, if we live in a primitive culture and believe that moonlight exerts an evil influence, we may over- or underestimate its brightness. Similarly, an adolescent couple trying to walk undetected in their neighborhood at night may overestimate the moon's brightness. Conversely, their curious neighbors may underestimate its brightness.

More relevant to the present discussion is the way in which non-visual information can affect visual perception. The apparent brightness of an object can be altered if the perceiver experiences intense pain, loses vestibular cues (and a corresponding sense of balance), becomes paralyzed, or even hears a loud noise. The point that modern-day perceptual researchers emphasize is that we simultaneously rely on all of our perceptual systems in making sense of any visual array.

The role of attention. How do individuals first notice and attend to internal physical sensations as opposed to external visual cues? Given that individuals can process only a finite amount of information at any given time, we have proposed that internal sensory and external environmental cues compete for attention (Pennebaker 1982). As the number and salience of external cues increase, attention to internal stimuli will necessarily decrease, and vice versa. When the environment lacks meaningful external information (such as when people engage in boring or tedious tasks), attention will tend to focus more internally, thereby causing an increase in symptom reporting. Thus, people should perceive and report more symptoms in unstimulating environments than in interesting ones.

A great deal of research now supports this competition-of-cues model. Various experiments demonstrate that people report higher levels of fatigue (Fillingim and Fine 1986; Pennebaker and Lightner 1980), increased heart palpitations (Pennebaker 1981), and even increased coughing (Pennebaker 1980) in boring situations than in stimulating ones. Manipulations that heighten self-attention also increase physical sympton reporting (Duval and Wicklund 1972; Mechanic 1980; Pennebaker and Brittingham 1982; Wegner and Guiliano 1980). Indeed, epidemiologic studies indicate that symptom reporting is elevated when individuals live alone or in rural environments, or work in undemanding or unstimulating settings (Moos and Van Dort 1977; National Center for Health Statistics 1980; Wan 1976). Conversely, increased focus of attention to the body heightens symptom reporting. It is noteworthy, however, that this increased symptom reporting is unrelated to accuracy of perceiving physiological change (Pennebaker and Watson 1988a).

The selective search for information. Another line of research is based on the assumption that organisms actively search their environment for information that will enable them to behave more adaptively (Neisser 1976). This scanning is not random but, rather, is guided by beliefs or mental sets that direct the ways in which information is sought and ultimately found. This principle is also relevant to the formation of health complaints. That is, health-related beliefs influence how people attend to and interpret bodily sensations (Pennebaker and Skelton 1981; Pennebaker and Watson 1988b).

Dramatic examples of the power of health beliefs, or schemas, can be seen in cases of "medical student's disease" and mass psychogenic illness. Regarding the former, approximately 70% of first-year medical students report symptoms of the diseases that they are studying (Woods et al. 1978). The students, who are undoubtedly under stress from sleep deprivation, exams, or other factors, can detect a number of subtle bodily sensations that probably reflect heightened autonomic activity. When they read about various obscure illnesses associated with ambiguous symptoms, the students then scrutinize their bodies particularly closely. Their disease beliefs or schemas direct the ways they attend to their bodies and interpret their symptoms.

Schemas and selective search also play an important role in cases of mass psychogenic illness (Colligan et al. 1982). In this illness large groups of individuals who typically work together report a related set of physical symptoms that have no clear organic basis. Mass psychogenic illness usually develops when one person in a setting becomes overtly sick and displays observable symptoms such as vomiting or fainting. These symptoms affect the belief processes of others in the setting—especially friends—who consequently experience similar, but less dramatic symptoms such as feelings of nausea or dizziness.

The perceptual approach is important in clarifying how healthy individuals typically detect and report symptoms in the real world. Obviously, the symptom-reporting process can also be exaggerated or dampened by rewards or punishments or by other forms of primary and secondary gains (Mechanic 1978). Most of our research on symptom reporting has been conducted on individuals who would not be classified as suffering from any of the somatoform disorders. Nevertheless, it is easy to see how extreme variants of these same processes could lead to the greatly magnified symptom reporting that characterizes these disorders. Indeed, somatization disorder and, to a lesser extent, hypochondriasis appear to be classic instances of individuals becoming hypervigilant about largely subtle and benign sensations.

Gender differences in information processing. An interesting outgrowth of our research on symptom perception has been the emergence of a consistent sex difference in how individuals notice, define, and react to symptoms. Specifically, women are particularly sensitive to external environmental cues and men to internal physiological cues in defining their symptoms. This conclusion is based on laboratory and field studies that have attempted to learn how accurately individuals perceive specific physiological activity.

Across virtually all highly controlled laboratory studies, men are consistently better able than women to detect heart rate (Katkin et al. 1981), stomach activity (Whitehead and Drescher 1980), blood pressure (Pennebaker et al. 1982), and blood glucose levels (Cox et al. 1985). In naturalistic field studies, however, both women and men are equally good at estimating blood pressure and blood glucose. (T. A. Roberts and J. W. Pennebaker, 1989, unpublished observations).

In a particularly strong test of this latter finding, a group of 19 diabetic patients who had had experience monitoring their blood glucose levels participated in a two-phase study in the hospital and, later, at home. In the hospital phase of the experiment, the subjects' glucose levels were directly manipulated over the course of a day—that is, a machine that simulated the activity of the pancreas took each patient on a blood glucose "roller-coaster ride" over the 8-hour experiment. Once every 10 minutes, subjects estimated their glucose levels. Overall, the correlations between actual and estimated blood glucose were .42 for men and .13 for women. Later, the same subjects estimated and measured their glucose levels several times each day for 2 weeks at home during their typical days. At home, where a variety of situational cues were present, the correlations between actual and estimated blood glucose were .58 for men and .69 for women.

Situational cues—such as time of day, room temperature, and so forth—are usually redundant with internal physiological cues. In other words, we can make fairly accurate educated guesses about people's physiological activity if we know the settings they are in. What is interesting, however, is that men and women differentially rely on internal versus external cues in defining the symptoms that they are feeling.

The use of different perceptual strategies by men and women may explain the large gender differences in somatization disorder, but not hypochondriasis (see Robbins and Kirmayer, Chapter 6, this volume). Given that women are especially sensitive to situational cues, their symptom-reporting patterns should reflect the settings that they are perceiving as stressful. Men, however, will tend to ignore the settings and focus on their physiological cues. Symptom reporting, then, will tend to mirror situational fluctations in women and physiological changes in men. Interestingly, hypochondriasis should not necessarily be gender linked, since it is not a disorder of symptom reporting per se.

Note that the gender difference in the perceptual bases of symptom reporting has been found in generally healthy individuals. Further, the effects are moderately strong but not overwhelming. At this point, the findings and explanations are intriguing and worthy of future study.

Dispositional Bases of Somatization: The Role of Negative Affectivity

Within the last few years, we and others have begun to examine the role that personality variables play in the formation and reporting of physical symptoms (Costa and McCrae 1987; Watson and Pennebaker 1989). Most of this research has centered on a mood-based disposition we call "negative affectivity" or trait NA. In our work, we have also examined a second mood disposition, which we have variously called "positive affectivity" or trait PA. Trait NA is essentially identical to several other dispositional constructs such as neuroticism, trait anxiety, pessimism (versus optimism), general maladjustment, and so on. In contrast, trait PA is strongly associated with extraversion and general energy or activation. It should be emphasized that the trait of positive affectivity is more associated with activity level and is *not* synonymous with happiness.

Trait NA reflects pervasive individual differences in negative mood and self-concept (Watson and Clark 1984). Individuals with high NA experience consistently higher levels of distress and dissatisfaction over time across different situations. High NA subjects are also more introspective and tend to dwell differentially on their failures and shortcomings. They tend to be negativistic, focusing on the negative aspects of themselves and others.

A great number of NA scales are available in the personality literature (Byrne 1961; Taylor 1953; Watson et al. 1988). In our own research on symptom reporting, we have relied primarily on two measures: the Negative Emotionality (Nem) Scale from Tellegen's Multiple Personality Questionnaire (Tellegen, in press), and the "general" or trait version of the NA scale from the Positive and Negative Affectivity Scales (PANAS) (Watson et al. 1988). Both of these scales assess the extent to which individuals report feeling scared, guilty, irritable, distressed, worried, and so forth. Similar to other trait NA measures, both scales are highly homogeneous and stable over time. For example, across several large samples consisting of both healthy adults and college students, the Nem scale had a mean coefficient alpha of .82 and a 12-week retest reliability of .72 (Tellegen, in press). Similarly, the trait NA scale from the PANAS is both internally consistent (coefficient alpha = .87) and strongly stable (8-week retest r = .71) (Watson et al. 1988).

Recently, we reviewed a large number of studies indicating that trait NA is highly correlated with virtually all measures of symptom reporting (Watson and Pennebaker 1989; Watson et al. 1988). Across several samples, using different NA scales and various measures of symptom reporting, NA markers had correlations typically in the .30 to .50 range with symptom reports, with a mean coefficient of approximately .40. Interestingly, high NA individuals consistently report all types of sensations and physical symptoms to a greater degree than do low NA individuals—even though high and low NA subjects do not differ noticeably on various objective health markers.

The reliable link between NA and symptom reporting, in the absence of any NA-related differences in objective health status, leads us to conclude that symptom reporting is strongly affected by the NA trait. High NA individuals appear to be hypervigilant about their bodies and have a lower threshold for noticing and reporting subtle bodily sensations. Because of their generally pessimistic view of the world, they are also most likely to worry about the implications of their perceived symptoms. In short, subjects with high NA would seem to be at greater risk for somatization disorder and, perhaps, hypochondriasis.

The importance of the link between NA and the somatoform disorders cannot be overemphasized. First, consistent with other aspects of the trait, high NA individuals will be more likely than others to report symptoms across all situations and over long time intervals. Because of this, excessive symptom reporting is not only influenced by transient situational stressors, but also reflects a stable personality trait. Second, reliance on symptom reports without a concurrent measure of NA can lead to a distorted view of the meaning and significance of these symptoms. As discussed in the final section of this chapter, it is critical that researchers and clinicians consider NA as a nuisance factor that must be assessed when trying to evaluate and treat reports of symptoms.

The Genetic Bases of Symptom Reporting

As discussed above, symptom reporting is influenced both by situational cues and by broad dispositional differences in distress and complaining. Closely allied with this evidence is recent work suggesting that the tendency to report symptoms and negative affect is strongly heritable. The genetic argument reflects common assumptions about the phenotypic bases of physiological functioning as well as recent findings concerning the inheritance of perceptual and emotional styles.

The awareness and reporting of physical symptoms depends, to a large degree, on the way information is processed in different parts of the brain. The somatosensory cortex, for example, fundamentally affects how individuals perceive sensations in their bodies. Beyond basic perception, the ability to report symptoms is dependent on the proper functioning of the language centers in the temporal and parietal lobes (Luria 1980). Further, it is well documented that central nervous system structure and function are, in turn, strongly genetically determined. Monozygotic twins, for example, have remarkably similar—albeit not identical—cortical structures, neurotransmitter activity, and electroencephalographic and autonomic nervous system activation compared with dizygotic twins (Lykken 1982). In short, the brain's biological hardware that underlies symptom perception clearly has a heritable basis.

Of particular relevance are a series of discoveries pointing to the genetic bases of personality dispositions and their associated cognitive, perceptual, and behavioral styles. Of greatest relevance are the findings of Tellegen and his colleagues at the University of Minnesota (Tellegen et al. 1988), who have conducted a large-scale examination of the heritability of trait NA. The Minnesota researchers investigated over 400 pairs of identical and fraternal twins who were reared either together or apart. Trait NA was assessed using a higher-order factor score from the Multidimensional Personality Questionnaire (Tellegen, in press). Overall, an estimated 55% of the variance on trait NA could be attributed to genetic factors, whereas only 2% was due to the shared familial environment. The remaining 43% of the variance is presumably attributable to measurement error and idiosyncratic situational influences that were not assessed by the researchers. A number of other large-scale studies have now reported similar findings in regard to the heritability of trait NA (Floderus-Myrhed et al. 1980; Fulker 1981; Pederson et al. 1988; Rose et al. 1988).

Unfortunately, the Minnesota project did not directly examine the heritability of symptom reporting. Nevertheless, the heritability of the NA trait strongly suggests that individuals' proclivity to report symptoms and sensations has a similar genetic basis. Given the currently available data, however, it is impossible to point with any certainty to the biological and/or psychological mechanisms underlying the genetics of somatization. Perhaps the most promising hypothesis links attentional vigilance with specific physiological substrates.

Jeffrey Gray (1982) points to the importance of inhibitory centers within the brain (such as those in the septum and hippocampus) as influencing—both directly and indirectly—individual differences in trait NA. When these inhibitory centers are activated, individuals become hypervigilant about the presence of novel stimuli in the environment. Gray believes that high NA subjects, whom he calls "trait anxious," have overactive inhibitory centers that result in their being characterologically hypervigilant. This hypervigilance probably affects symptom reporting in two ways. First, subjects with high NA should be more attentive to subtle sensations in their bodies. Second, because their scanning is fraught with anxiety and uncertainty, high NA individuals may be more likely to interpret minor symptoms and sensations as painful or pathological.

Interestingly, Barsky and his colleagues (Barsky and Klerman 1983) also argue that hypervigilance, selective attention, and the tendency to view somatic sensations as ominous are all important elements in the amplification of symptoms. Thus, the perceptual style of individuals with high NA may be largely responsible for their enhanced somatic complaining.

IMPLICATIONS FOR FUTURE SOMATIZATION RESEARCH

The previous sections of this chapter have focused on the perceptual, dispositional, and genetic bases of symptom reporting. Given that physical symptom reports reflect more than biological activity, the research on somatic symptoms raises some questions about future somatization research and theory. In this section we first raise the issue whether the somatoform disorders should be reclassified as personality disorders rather than as Axis I diagnoses. We then address the potential problem of NA as a nuisance factor in somatization research. Finally, we propose that more studies in the future employ repeated measures or within-subject designs in attempts to better understand somatization.

Rethinking the DSM Classification of Somatoform Disorders

As the dispositional and genetic research suggests, the tendency to notice, report, and worry about physical symptoms undoubtedly reflects an enduring trait or group of traits. In this context, it is not surprising that symptom reporting is similarly stable and traitlike over time (Pennebaker 1982; Watson and Pennebaker 1989).

These results have important implications for understanding and classifying the somatoform disorders. Of these disorders, somatization disorder and hypochondriasis appear to have the clearest links to measures of NA. It is not coincidental, then, that one of the defining characteristics of somatization disorder, according to the *Diagnostic and Statistical Manual of Mental Disorders*, Third Edition, Revised (DSM-III-R), is "a history of many physical complaints . . . beginning before the age of 30 and persisting for several years" (American Psychiatric Association 1987, p. 263). Similarly, hypochondriasis is listed as having a course that is usually chronic, with some degree of waxing and waning of symptoms.

Given the chronic and enduring nature of these somatoform disorders, it makes sense to reconsider their current status as Axis I problems within the DSM framework. Rather than reflecting temporary behaviors associated with psychosocial stressors, somatization disorder and hypochondriasis appear to be dispositionally based syndromes more in line with the definition of personality disorders. Clearly, however, additional longitudinal and/or twin data must be collected before the optimal nosological placement of these somatoform disorders can be firmly established.

Disentangling Negative Affectivity From Symptom Reporting

Another implication of our approach is that, in many cases,

heightened symptom reporting may reflect elevated NA levels rather than actual changes in physiological activity. To truly understand symptom reporting, then, it is important to statistically control for trait NA. In other words, NA can be expected to act as a general nuisance factor in health research, one that taps psychologically important but organically spurious variance in physical symptom measures. As we have discussed elsewhere (Watson and Pennebaker 1989), there is an inherent problem in any study that uses a health complaint scale as its criterion for health and that includes, as a psychological predictor, a measure with a subjective distress component. The danger always exists that such a predictor is assessing variance that is uninteresting from an objective health standpoint.

A good example of this problem can be seen in the often-reported finding that measures of perceived stress (e.g., major life changes, daily hassles) correlate significantly with self-reported health complaints. Such results are usually taken to mean that elevated stress levels cause illness and other health problems. This interpretation is complicated, however, by the fact that perceived stress measures have been found to have a substantial subjective distress component that correlates with NA. It therefore seems likely that stress-symptom correlations partly reflect their overlapping NA component. Indeed, we have found this to be true with a variety of samples (Watson and Pennebaker 1989; Watson and Pennebaker, in press).

A clear implication of these findings is that future research on symptom reporting should also collect concurrent self-reports of NA. By using simple covariation or multiple regression procedures, researchers can get a better estimate of the influence of this trait, especially when any causal mechanisms are being considered.

Between-Subjects Versus Within-Subject Designs

A final issue concerns the research designs that symptom researchers employ. Many health investigators continue to use strict between-subjects designs, wherein large numbers of respondents are assessed on a single occasion. Because such designs are based solely on interindividual variability, they allow individual difference variables, such as trait NA, to confound the results, thereby producing data that may be uninterpretable.

Given that trait NA invariably influences overall levels of health complaints, perceived stress, and many other variables, health researchers would be wise to make greater use of within-subject designs that focus on intraindividual changes in symptom reporting over time and across different situations. People typically visit physicians, for example, when they note a significant *change* in symptom levels.

Medication use, restriction of daily activities, and other self-initiated health behaviors are also based on perceived changes in body state (Pennebaker 1982).

That health-related behaviors are guided to a large degree by changes in perceived symptoms helps to explain why trait NA is apparently unrelated to health-care utilization and other health-related behaviors (Watson and Pennebaker 1989). Because trait NA is virtually synonymous with subjective distress, our conclusions are superficially inconsistent with the sizable literature showing that highly distressed individuals make extensive use of medical facilities for both physical and psychological reasons (Escobar et al. 1989; Katon 1984; Katon et al. 1984). Trait NA, however, is related to stable individual differences in symptom level. As noted above, illness-related behaviors are likely to be more affected by perceived changes in symptoms than by the absolute level of symptomatology per se.

The problem of self-reports and dispositions is nicely illustrated by two undergraduates who assisted in our research. In the year that they worked for us, one student always reported aches, pains, fatigue, and assorted symptoms, whereas the other never noted any symptoms or sensations. During the year, both had a single illness episode associated with high fever and vomiting for which they visited a physician. During this illness, both students reported symptoms that were far above their baseline levels of complaining. Within weeks of the illness, however, both students returned to their pre-illness symptom-reporting rates.

The point of this story is to demonstrate that symptom reports can be useful. Indeed, they can be predictive of both internal physiological activity and behavior change. We again emphasize, however, that symptom reports will prove most valuable when viewed from the context of within-subject designs, wherein researchers can detect symptom change rather than simply symptom level. We should also note that between-subjects and within-subject designs are not mutually exclusive. Indeed, combining the two in a single study can produce heuristically powerful results (Pennebaker 1990; Pennebaker and Epstein 1983; Watson 1988) in which both intraindividual symptom change and interindividual symptom levels can be examined. Failing to consider the central role of NA in between-subjects research, however, will produce studies that add little to our understanding of health.

REFERENCES

American Psychiatric Association: Diagnostic and Statistical Manual of Mental Disorders, 3rd Edition, Revised. Washington, DC, American Psychiatric Association, 1987

Barsky AJ, Klerman GL: Overview: hypochondriasis, bodily complaints, and somatic styles. Am J Psychiatry 140:273–283, 1983

Boring EG: A History of Experimental Psychology. New York, Appleton-Century-Crofts, 1950

Byrne D: The Repression-Sensitization Scale: rationale, reliability, and validity. J Pers 29:334–349, 1961

Colligan MJ, Pennebaker JW, Murphy LR: Mass Psychogenic Illness: A Social Psychological Analysis. Hillsdale, NJ, Erlbaum, 1982

Costa PT Jr, McCrae RR: Neuroticism, somatic complaints, and disease: is the bark worse than the bite? J Pers 55:299–316, 1987

Cox DJ, Clark WL, Gonder-Frederick LA, et al: Accuracy of perceiving blood glucose in IDDM. Diabetes Care 8:529–535, 1985

Duval S, Wicklund RA: A Theory of Objective Self-Awareness. New York, Academic, 1972

Escobar JL, Rubio-Stipec M, Canino G, et al: Somatic Symptom Index (SSI): a new and abridged somatization construct: prevalence and epidemiological correlates in two large community samples. J Nerv Ment Dis 177:140–146, 1989

Fillingim RB, Fine MA: The effects of internal versus external information processing on symptom perception in an exercise setting. Health Psychol 5:115–123, 1986

Floderus-Myrhed B, Pedersen N, Rasmuson I: Assessment of heritability for personality based on a short-form Eysenck Personality Inventory: a study of 12,898 twin pairs. Behav Genet 10:153–161, 1980

Fulker DW: The genetic and environmental architecture of psychoticism, extraversion, and neuroticism, in A Model for Personality. Edited by Eysenck HJ. New York, Springer-Verlag, 1981, pp 88–122

Gibson JJ: The Ecological Approach to Visual Perception. Boston, MA, Houghton-Mifflin, 1979

Gray JA: The Neuropsychology of Anxiety: An Enquiry into the Functions of the Septo-Hippocampal System. New York, Oxford University Press, 1982

Katkin ES, Blascovich J, Goldband S: Empirical assessment of visceral self-perception: individual and sex differences in the acquisition of heartbeat discrimination. J Pers Soc Psychol 40:1095–1101, 1981

Katon W: Depression: relationship to somatization and chronic medical illness. J Clin Psychiatry 45:4–12, 1984

Katon W, Ries R, Kleinman A: The prevalence of somatization in primary care. Compr Psychiatry 25:208–215, 1984

Lipowski ZJ: Somatization: the concept and its application. Am J Psychiatry 145:1358–1368, 1988

Luria AR: Higher Cortical Functions in Man. New York, Basic Books, 1980

Lykken DT: Research with twins: the concept of emergenesis. Psychophysiology 19:361–373, 1982

Mechanic D: Medical Sociology, 2nd Edition. New York, Free Press, 1978

Mechanic D: The experience and reporting of common physical complaints. J Health Soc Behav 21:146–155, 1980

Moos R, Van Dort B: Physical and emotional symptoms and campus health center utilization. Soc Psychiatry 12:107–115, 1977

National Center for Health Statistics: Basic data on depressive symptomatology (ser 11, no 216). Washington, DC, U.S. Government Printing Office, 1980

Neisser U: Cognition and Reality. San Francisco, CA, WH Freeman, 1976

Pederson NL, Plomin R, McClearn GE, et al: Neuroticism, extraversion, and related traits in adult twins reared apart and reared together. J Pers Soc Psychol 55:950–957, 1988

Pennebaker JW: Perceptual and environmental determinants of coughing. Basic and Applied Social Psychology 1:83–91, 1980

Pennebaker JW: Stimulus characteristics influencing estimation of heart rate. Psychophysiology 18:540–548, 1981

Pennebaker JW: The Psychology of Physical Symptoms. New York, Springer-Verlag, 1982

Pennebaker JW: Opening Up: The Healing Power of Confiding in Others. New York, William Morrow, 1990

Pennebaker JW, Brittingham GL: Environmental and sensory cues affecting the perception of physical symptoms, in Advances in Environmental Psychology, Vol 4. Edited by Baum A, Singer J. Hillsdale, NJ, Erlbaum, 1982, pp 115–136

Pennebaker JW, Epstein D: Implicit psychophysiology: effects of common beliefs and idiosyncratic physiological responses on symptom reporting. J Pers 51:468–496, 1983

Pennebaker JW, Lightner JM: Competition of internal and external information in an exercise setting. J Pers Soc Psychol 39:165–174, 1980

Pennebaker JW, Skelton JA: Selective monitoring of bodily sensations. J Pers Soc Psychol 41:213–223, 1981

Pennebaker JW, Watson D: Blood pressure estimation and beliefs among normotensives and hypertensives. Health Psychol 7:309–328, 1988a

Pennebaker JW, Watson D: Self-reports and physiological measures in the workplace, in Occupational Stress: Issues and Developments in Research. Edited by Hurrel JJ, Murphy LR, Sauter SL, et al. Philadelphia, PA, Taylor and Francis, 1988b, pp 184–199

Pennebaker JW, Gonder-Frederick LA, Stewart H, et al: Physical symptoms associated with blood pressure. Psychophysiology 19:201–210, 1982

Robbins JM, Kirmayer LJ: Illness cognition, symptom reporting and somatization in primary care, in Illness Behavior: A Multidisciplinary Model. Edited by McHugh S, Vallis TM. New York, Plenum, 1986, pp 283–302

Rose RJ, Koskenvuo M, Kaprio J, et al: Shared genes, shared experiences, and similarity of personality: data from 14,288 adult Finnish co-twins. J Pers Soc Psychol 54:161–171, 1988

Taylor JA: A personality scale of manifest anxiety. Journal of Abnormal and Social Psychology 48:285–290, 1953

Tellegen A: Multidimensional Personality Questionnaire. Minneapolis, MN, University of Minnesota Press (in press)

Tellegen A, Lykken DT, Bouchard TJ Jr, et al: Personality similarity in twins reared apart and together. J Pers Soc Psychol 54:1031–1039, 1988

Wan T: Predicting self-assessed health status: a multivariate approach. Health Serv Res 11:464–477, 1976

Watson D: The vicissitudes of mood measurement: effects of varying descriptors, time frames, and response formats on measures of positive and negative affect. J Pers Soc Psychol 55:128–141, 1988

Watson D, Clark LA: Negative affectivity: The disposition to experience aversive emotional states. Psychol Bull 96:465–490, 1984

Watson D, Pennebaker JW: Health complaints, stress, and distress: exploring the central role of negative affectivity. Psychol Rev 96:234–254, 1989

Watson D, Pennebaker JW: Situational, dispositional, and genetic basis of symptom reporting, in Mental Representations in Health and Illness. Edited by Skelton JA, Croyle RT. New York, Springer-Verlag (in press)

Watson D, Clark LA, Tellegen A: Development and validation of brief measures of positive and negative affect: the PANAS Scales. J Pers Soc Psychol 54:1063–1070, 1988

Wegner DM, Guiliano T: Arousal-induced attention to self. J Pers Soc Psychol 38:719–726, 1980

Whitehead WE, Drescher VM: Perception of gastric contractions and self-control of gastric motility. Psychophysiology 17:552–558, 1980

Woods S, Natterson J, Silverman J: Medical students' disease: hypochondriasis in medical education. J Med Educ 41:785–790, 1978

Chapter 3

Somatization and Psychiatric Disorders

Gregory E. Simon, M.D.

One hundred years ago the puzzle of somatization inspired Freud and Breuer to develop the concepts of unconscious conflict, defenses, and resistances that have shaped much of contemporary psychiatry. The unexplained physical symptoms of those Victorian "somatizers" were considered outward signs of more significant underlying psychological disturbances. Patients' continued insistence on the physical nature of their symptoms was seen as a defense against these underlying psychiatric causes. Psychoanalysis and the rest of psychiatry eventually shifted emphasis away from physical symptoms to those psychiatric disorders presumed to cause hysteria or somatization. The subsequent 100 years of progress in psychiatry have included dramatic advances in our understanding and treatment of those more conventional mental disorders. Our understanding of the process of somatization, however, sometimes appears to have progressed little since the 1890s.

Somatizing patients continue to respond to our psychological explanations with skepticism and frustration. Whether we attempt to understand their unexplained physical symptoms as manifestations of unconscious conflict, family dysfunction, habitual behavior patterns, or perturbed neurotransmitters, our patients often feel that we do not understand them at all. Clinicians familiar with somatizing patients can readily recall the therapeutic impasses that result from this feeling of misunderstanding. Our patients also regard much of the expanding research on somatization as being similarly misguided. Publications of support organizations for patients with myalgic encephalitis (Myalgic Encephalomyelitis Society 1985) and chronic fatigue syndrome (Jackson 1988) contain criticism of research linking these conditions to depression and psychological distress. Like Freud's hysterical patients, our patients with unexplained physical symptoms regard our

This chapter was written while the author was a Robert Wood Johnson Clinical Scholar at the University of Washington, Seattle, Washington.

clinical and scientific efforts as unhelpful. From this we might conclude either that the psychological defenses of somatizing patients are impervious to 100 years of interpretation or that our patients might know something that we do not.

In this chapter I use the term *somatization* to refer to the persistent tendency shown by some patients to present with functional somatic distress or physical symptoms that have no apparent medical explanation. Briquet's syndrome and its offspring, somatization disorder (American Psychiatric Association 1987), are presumed to represent the most extreme version of this tendency. Escobar and colleagues (1987a) have developed a more inclusive standard for somatization that identifies approximately 5% of the general population as having the greatest tendency toward reporting of unexplained symptoms.

Hypochondriasis and somatization may often coexist, but this presentation will define them more distinctly than their overlap in clinical situations might suggest. Such a distinction is consistent with the standards of DSM-III-R (American Psychiatric Association 1987). Hypochondriasis is characterized by particular thoughts or ideas: morbid fear of illness and belief that one suffers from some undiagnosed disease. In contrast, somatization is characterized by physical symptoms and unpleasant bodily sensations. Although hypochondriasis and somatization may overlap, the former definition focuses on cognition and the latter on perception.

Most definitions of somatization include the assumption that unexplained physical symptoms result from latent psychological distress (Barsky and Klerman 1983; Kaplan et al. 1988; Katon et al. 1982; Kellner 1985). The use of the term *somatization* implies that there is some underlying process that is being somatized. The DSM-III-R description of somatoform disorders notes as one of the central features "positive evidence, or a strong presumption, that the symptoms are linked to psychological factors or conflicts" (American Psychiatric Association 1987, p. 255). This presumption about mechanism or cause is unusual among the avowedly atheoretical descriptions of DSM-III-R, and the reference to hidden psychodynamic processes is unique.

All descriptions of the process of somatization contain three main components. First, somatizing patients report physical symptoms for which medical evaluation reveals no apparent cause. Second, these physical symptoms usually accompany psychiatric symptoms or psychological distress. Third, somatizing patients are frequent users of medical care.

In this chapter I will examine recent research on somatization in an attempt to determine what, if anything, is being somatized. I will first consider data on the relationships among the three factors described above: physical symptom reporting, psychiatric disorder, and health care utilization. Next, I will consider possible models to explain the apparent strong associations between these factors. Potential research techniques for clarifying the relationship between somatization and psychiatric disorder will also be considered. Finally, the clinical implications of various models for somatization will be discussed.

PSYCHIATRIC DISORDERS, SOMATIC SYMPTOMS, AND HEALTH CARE UTILIZATION

Psychiatric Disorders and Health Care Utilization

Of the interrelationships described above, the first examined is that between psychiatric disorders and the use of health care services. Previous investigations have clearly demonstrated a strong association. Typically, these studies have focused on the prevalence of psychiatric diagnosis among medical service users. Nielsen and Williams (1980) used the Beck Depression Inventory to study the prevalence of depression among a consecutive sample of medical clinic patients. They found that 12.2% of these patients met criteria for depression of at least mild severity. Jones and colleagues (1987) studied patients of family-practice residents using a self-report measure of psychological distress, the General Health Questionnaire (GHQ), followed by a structured psychiatric interview, the National Institute of Mental Health (NIMH) Diagnostic Interview Schedule (DIS), for subjects with elevated GHQ scores. Of 139 patients screened, 42 had at least one DIS psychiatric diagnosis within the previous year. Von Korff and colleagues (1987) administered both the GHQ and the DIS to 809 patients of an urban primary-care teaching clinic. Using the GHQ they identified 30% of the patients as having a psychiatric disorder, while using the DIS they identified 8% as having an anxiety or depressive disorder within the previous month. Kessler and colleagues (1985) used the GHQ to screen adult patients in a rural multispecialty clinic. A sample of subjects stratified according to GHQ scores was then studied on two occasions 6 months apart using a structured diagnostic interview, the Schedule for Affective Disorders and Schizophrenia–Lifetime Version (SADS-L). Approximately 35% of the subjects met criteria for one or more SADS diagnoses on one or more of the interviews. Depressive and anxiety disorders accounted for the bulk of cases. Barrett and colleagues (1988) used a self-report depression questionnaire to screen primary-care clinic patients for a subsequent SADS interview. They found a 27% prevalence of current psychiatric disorder based on

Research Diagnostic Criteria (RDC). Depressive and anxiety disorders dominated; however, the diagnostic interview focused specifically on these two categories. Other reports describe similar frequencies of self-reported psychological distress and psychiatric diagnoses in medical settings (Hankin and Locke 1982; Schulberg et al. 1987).

These studies appear to consistently demonstrate high levels of psychiatric symptomatology and psychiatric diagnoses among medical patients. Self-report screening instruments assessing psychological distress in general, or depressive symptoms in particular, consistently identify 20% to 30% of medical patients as "cases." Structured interviews typically find that 10% to 20% of primary care outpatients meet criteria for current depressive and/or anxiety disorders. This prevalence is two to three times higher than that measured in the general population using similar instruments (Regier et al. 1988). Increased use of medical care, however, may not be specifically linked to anxiety or depression. Studies of psychiatric disorder in medical settings typically focus on more common diagnoses and exclude examination of others. Sample sizes are often not sufficient to detect significant increases in the rates of less common psychiatric disorders. Medical service users could demonstrate as much as a fivefold increase in prevalence of less common disorders such as schizophrenia or mania, and such an association could go undetected by the studies described above.

Population-based data also support the association between medical service use and psychiatric diagnosis. Kessler and colleagues (1987) note that respondents in the NIMH Epidemiologic Catchment Area (ECA) study who reported use of outpatient health services in the preceding 6 months had higher rates of DIS psychiatric diagnoses during the subsequent 6 months than did nonusers of health services (21% vs. 16%). Anxiety and depressive disorders were clearly more prevalent among medical patients. Schizophrenic disorders showed a similar increased prevalence, but baseline rates of schizophrenia were low enough to preclude any confident judgment about an association between psychosis and medical service use. Substance use and abuse diagnoses were the most common in both groups, but did not show a clear pattern of increase among users of medical services.

Surveys of patients and providers suggest that psychiatric disorders account for a significant portion of outpatient health care utilization. Data from the 1981 National Ambulatory Medical Care Survey (Schurman et al. 1985) demonstrate that 8% of all visits to non-psychiatric primary care physicians result in a psychiatric diagnosis. Reporting on a survey of minor psychiatric morbidity and medical care use in over 3,000 London residents, Williams and colleagues

(1986) concluded that approximately 20% of primary care visits could be attributed to psychiatric distress. Stewart and colleagues (1975) studied 389 family-practice visits and concluded that overt or covert psychosocial problems were the reasons for consultation in approximately one-third of the cases.

Functional Somatic Symptoms and Use of Medical Care

The second relationship examined is that between unexplained physical symptoms and the use of health services. Data, here, also demonstrate a strong association. Escobar and colleagues (1987b) have reported on evidence from the Los Angeles sample of the ECA study. Respondents meeting criteria for Escobar's abridged somatization construct more often reported recent use of medical services than did nonsomatizing individuals. Swartz and colleagues (1987) found that ECA respondents meeting full DSM-III criteria (American Psychiatric Association 1980) for somatization disorder used outpatient medical services approximately three times as often as other respondents. Smith and colleagues (1986) studied health care utilization by 41 patients meeting DSM-III criteria for somatization disorder. These patients with the most severe form of somatization used inpatient and outpatient services at a rate 10 times that of the United States population. Zoccolillo and Cloninger (1986) found that 50 women with somatization disorder had three times as many hospitalizations and surgeries as did a comparison group with major depression.

Functional Somatic Symptoms and Psychiatric Disorders

The third link in this triangle involving functional somatic symptoms, psychiatric disorders, and the use of health care is that between unexplained physical symptoms and psychiatric symptomatology. Escobar and colleagues (1987a) have reported data from the Los Angeles sample of the ECA study demonstrating an association between somatization symptoms and diagnosis of depression or dysthymia. Review of data from all sites shows a strong association between somatization symptoms and psychiatric symptoms across all diagnoses (Simon 1990).

Studies of patients reporting specific types of unexplained physical symptoms demonstrate a clear link between these somatization syndromes and psychiatric morbidity. These investigations typically use structured diagnostic interviews and self-report measures of psychiatric symptoms to compare patients presenting with particular unexplained symptoms with control groups of community residents or medically ill patients. Walker and colleagues (1988) used such a technique to demonstrate an increased rate of affective disorder and substance abuse in women seeking care for chronic pelvic pain. In an uncontrolled study of women undergoing hysterectomy for reasons other than cancer, Martin and colleagues (1977) found a 57% prevalence of psychiatric disorder. Sullivan et al. (1988) demonstrated an association between disabling tinnitus and affective disorder. Studies of patients with irritable bowel syndrome (Fossey et al. 1989; Young et al. 1976) report elevated rates of depression and anxiety disorders. Cormier and colleagues (1988) compared patients who had chest pain that was unexplained by cardiac diagnostic studies with chest-pain patients who had exercise tests or coronary arteriograms diagnostic of ischemic heart disease. The patients with unexplained symptoms demonstrated a markedly higher prevalence of depression, panic disorder, and phobias. The above studies, however, all examined patient groups that were self-selected or referred for treatment. Studies of functional somatic symptoms in nonpatient groups (to be discussed below) suggest that psychiatric disorders may be associated more with seeking care for functional symptoms than with the functional symptoms themselves.

These studies appear to show a consistent association between somatization and depression. Typically, somatization shows a stronger association to lifetime history of depression than to current diagnosis (Cormier et al. 1988; Sullivan et al. 1988; Walker et al. 1988). Some investigations also demonstrate an increased rate of anxiety disorders, but none have included enough subjects to reliably examine the frequency of less-common psychiatric diagnoses.

MODELS OF THE RELATIONSHIP BETWEEN SOMATIZATION AND PSYCHIATRIC DISORDERS

Review of the evidence discussed above suggests strong interrelationships among somatization, psychiatric disorders, and the use of health services. One might propose a variety of causal models to explain these observed relationships. Although these models are clearly not mutually exclusive, they will be discussed here separately for reasons of clarity. The causal schemes discussed probably all contribute to the process of somatization.

Somatization as a Psychological Defense

The traditional view explains that physical-symptom reporting and health-care seeking result from an altered presentation of psychiatric disorder, usually anxiety disorders or depression (Figure 3-1). This scheme is based on early psychoanalytic notions that considered hysterical symptoms as highly edited or transformed versions of forbidden unconscious impulses. Physical symptoms served the defensive function of allowing some expression of distress while keeping unacceptable wishes out of awareness. In the modern version, physical symptoms continue to function as defenses; they serve as expressions of distress that allow underlying depression or anxiety to remain out of awareness. Somatizing patients are said to preferentially express psychological distress through physical channels (Katon et al. 1982). Nemiah and Sifneos (Nemiah 1977) developed the concept of *alexithymia* to describe this group of patients who were thought to have "no words for feelings."

Empirical data suggest, however, that physical symptoms and

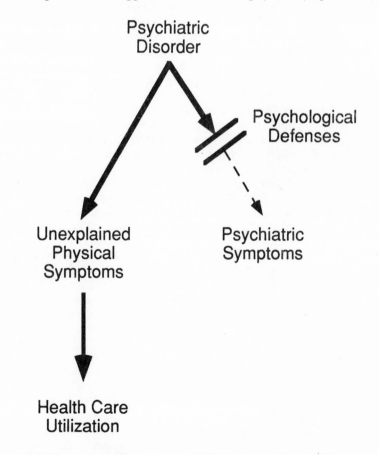

Figure 3-1. Somatization as a "masked" expression of psychiatric illness.

psychological symptoms are not alternative channels for expression of distress. Both types of symptoms typically occur together. If unexplained physical symptoms are intended to defend against awareness of psychological distress, they appear to serve that function poorly. Self-report symptom inventories typically show strong links between reporting of physical distress and psychological distress (Costa and McCrae 1980, 1985). Studies using the Cornell Medical Index (Imboden et al. 1961) and the Hopkins Symptom Checklist (G. E. Simon and W. Katon, 1989, unpublished data) with somatizing patients show high correlations between symptoms of somatization and psychological distress. In a study of menstrual symptoms among female medical students, Sherry et al. (1988) demonstrated a strong association between physical symptoms and self-reported psychological distress. Oxman et al. (1985) used linguistic analysis of the speech of somatizing patients to study the relationship between somatization and expressed emotional distress. These patients showed no apparent preference for discussion of bodily themes and no tendency to avoid discussion of negative emotions.

Although these findings give little support to the notion of alexithymia, they do not require that we abandon a model in which psychiatric disorder leads to somatization. Instead of considering unexplained physical symptoms as defenses against anxiety or depression, one might reasonably regard them as parallel expressions of distress. Studies of psychiatric patients demonstrate an association between psychiatric symptoms and somatic symptoms without medical explanation. Clancy and Noyes's (1976) classic description of panic disorder delineates the numerous physical symptoms and the accompanying medical care utilization of patients with anxiety disorders. Various studies of patients presenting with depressive symptoms have found high levels of physical-symptom reporting. Waxman and colleagues (1985) studied 127 community-dwelling older adults and found an association between depression assessed by the Geriatric Depression Scale and self-reported physical symptoms assessed by the Cornell Medical Index. This association persisted after adjustment for medical illness. Mathew and colleagues (1981) compared 51 drug-free depressed patients to age- and sex-matched control subjects. Depressed patients more frequently endorsed all 27 physical symptoms assessed, although none of the patients had any apparent chronic or acute medical conditions. These studies do not necessarily imply a specific association between somatization and depression or anxiety disorders. Examination of patients with other psychiatric diagnoses might yield similar findings. One study reported by Silver (1987), however, does describe higher levels of physical-symptom reporting among depressed inpatients than among inpatients with various other psychiatric diagnoses.

Somatization as a Nonspecific Amplification of Distress

A second model would explain elevated levels of both physical and psychiatric symptoms as consequences of nonspecific underlying distress (Figure 3-2). Patients who tend to perceive and report unpleasant sensations would be expected to endorse higher levels of all

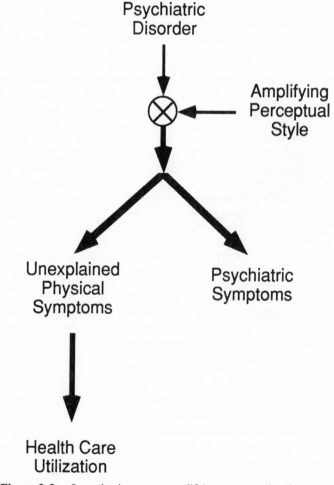

Figure 3-2. Somatization as an amplifying perceptual style.

types of symptoms. This tendency to experience aversive emotional states has been described by Watson and others (Watson and Clark 1984; Watson and Tellegen 1985) as "negative affectivity." Pennebaker and colleagues (1982; Pennebaker and Watson, Chapter 2, this volume) have conducted numerous investigations in college students and healthy volunteers, demonstrating the relationship between negative affective states and reporting of physical symptoms. They describe high symptom reporting as a personality trait influenced by experimental manipulations of psychological state (Pennebaker et al. 1977).

Balint's (1957) psychoanalytical investigations of emotional distress in primary care clinics led to similar conclusions. He coined the term "basic fault" to refer to defects in early development that led patients to experience generalized or nonspecific distress and to present to medical providers with both physical and emotional complaints.

These hypotheses view somatosensory amplification as a stable personality trait that influences processing of all sensory stimuli. Consequently, somatization is thought to result from an amplifying somatic style rather than from a specific psychiatric diagnosis.

Some previous research has examined the role of stable personality styles in sensory processing. Byrne (1964) has investigated the personality variable *repression-sensitization,* a measure of the tendency to focus on threatening or anxiety-provoking stimuli. In a study of college undergraduates (Byrne et al. 1968), sensitization was associated with more reported physical symptoms and greater use of health services. Studies of perceptual sensitivity demonstrated higher sensitivity to visual stimuli in hypochondriacal subjects than in control subjects (Hanback and Revelle 1978). Petrie (1978) proposed a common central mechanism that may augment or reduce sensory input and found a correlation between amplification of kinesthetic stimuli and augmentation of experimental pain. Buschbaum and Silverman (1968) operationalized this concept of a central augmenting or reducing process by measuring average electroencephalographic response evoked by visual stimuli. Augmentation of average evoked responses correlated with augmentation on a measure of kinesthetic perception. One study of auditory and visual perception, however, suggests that cortical augmentation or reduction of perception may be inconsistent across sensory modalities (Raine et al. 1981).

Building on this earlier work, Barsky (1979; Barsky et al. 1988b) has developed the concept of *somatosensory amplification* to explain the process by which psychological distress leads to physical-symptom sensitivity. All symptoms are thought of as beginning with peripheral sensation that leads to a cortical elaboration or reactive component. This reactive component may amplify or reduce the initial sensation. Aversive psychological states affect this system by increasing arousal and vigilance, thereby lowering the threshold for perceiving and reporting bodily events. Through this selective focus on noxious sensations, nonspecific distress is channeled into physical symptoms. This generalized amplification of bodily events results in the "diffuse positive review of systems" bemoaned by medical practitioners. Similarly, amplifying patients report higher levels of psychiatric symptoms as increased arousal results in a reduced threshold for perceiving and reporting emotional distress. Negative affect also increases pessimism, making patients more likely to attribute noxious bodily sensations to undiagnosed disease.

Recent research supports the clinical importance of somatosensory amplification in somatization. Barsky and colleagues (1988b) have developed a self-report measure of somatosensory amplification that can be used to inquire about sensitivity to various normal bodily events such as noise, temperature, blood flow, and intestinal peristalsis. The amplification scale has demonstrated good internal consistency and test-retest reliability in preliminary studies (Barsky et al. 1988b). In a study of symptom severity in upper respiratory infection (Barsky et al. 1988b), scores on the amplification scale correlated strongly with psychological symptoms assessed by the Hopkins Symptom Checklist–90 (SCL-90; Derogatis et al. 1973) and with self-reported physical symptoms. A study of symptom development among plastics workers following chemical exposure (Simon et al. 1990) found amplification scores to be a stronger predictor of unexplained physical symptoms than current psychiatric diagnosis assessed by the DIS or current psychiatric symptoms measured by the SCL-90.

One variation on the amplification hypothesis considers somatization as a consequence of abnormalities in the neuropsychology of information processing. Research in this area has typically examined patients with full somatization disorder. Meares and Horvath (1972) examined physiological responses to auditory stimulation in 16 patients with somatization disorder and found a failure of accommodation to repeated stimuli. Flor-Henry and colleagues (1981) demonstrated bifrontal abnormalities of neuropsychological testing of somatization disorder patients. They argued that somatization results from defects in processing and analysis of somatic signals. A review by Miller (1984) suggests that somatization results from a predominant right-hemisphere style of information processing. Von Knorring and Perris (1981) compared levels of various neurotransmitter metabolites in subjects demonstrating cortical augmentation or reduction of visual stimuli. They concluded that an augmenting sensory style is related to low activity in the serotonergic, dopaminergic, and endorphinergic pathways. Family studies demonstrating a heritable component of somatization (Bohman et al. 1984; Torgerson 1986) support the role of biologically determined abnormalities of perception. Buschbaum (1974) has studied familial patterns of information processing and demonstrated that visual and auditory EEG evoked potentials show greater similarity in identical twins than in fraternal twins. This greater concordance in identical twins suggests a heritable neurophysiological basis to augmentation or reduction of sensory stimuli.

Somatization and the Diagnostic Significance of Symptoms

The hypothesis that somatizing patients nonspecifically amplify both physical and psychological distress raises questions about the meaning of psychiatric symptoms in this group. Primary care practitioners traditionally discount many of the items endorsed in somatizing patients' diffusely positive symptom reviews. This process effectively adjusts physical symptom histories for these patients' tendency to overreport. Consideration of psychiatric-symptom reporting among somatizing patients usually makes no similar adjustment. Depression and anxiety are considered to have the same validity and diagnostic significance among patients who frequently report all types of symptoms as they do among patients who report psychiatric symptoms in isolation.

This differential treatment of physical and emotional symptoms results from factors unique to the process of psychiatric diagnosis. Medical diagnosis typically considers symptom reports to be imperfect and inconsistent indicators of underlying disease processes. We use initial symptom histories to guide the collection of other types of data, usually anatomic and physiological data collected through physical examination and laboratory tests. Through this process we can discover, for example, which patients presenting with chest pain have anatomic abnormalities of their coronary arteries that would appear to produce the symptoms. We conclude that patients without anatomic coronary artery abnormalities must have chest pain of a different type than patients with such findings, even though the symptom reports of both groups of patients may be identical. If we discover no evidence of underlying disease to account for a patient's reported symptoms, we consider the symptoms "functional" and conclude that such symptoms have very different meaning than do identical symptoms in patients with detectable organic disease. Psychiatric diagnosis allows no such distinction between functional and organic symptoms. Psychiatric diagnosticians typically have no sources of information other than symptom histories. Without any other data, we cannot consider whether reported psychiatric symptoms have the same diagnostic meaning in patients who endorse many symptoms of all types as they do in patients who endorse few symptoms. One exception to this description is illustrative. Although patients with somatization disorder may report hallucinations (American Psychiatric Association 1987), this symptom is not considered to have the same diagnostic meaning in this group as it would among psychiatric patients without such a tendency to overreport symptoms of all types.

The amplification model, therefore, has implications that differ significantly from those of the more traditional model discussed earlier. Somatization is thought to result from an amplifying style of information processing rather than from "masked" presentation of psychiatric disorder. Psychiatric symptoms in somatizing patients are considered as amplified expressions of underlying generalized distress that may not necessarily have specific diagnostic implications. Goldenberg (1989) has made such an argument concerning the reported high prevalence of depression in patients with fibromyalgia, a syndrome of unexplained fatigue, aching, and muscle tenderness. He points out that patients seeking care for fibromyalgia have been self-selected for high levels of physical-symptom reporting. Reporting of psychiatric symptoms, especially vegetative symptoms such as fatigue or appetite disturbance, may not imply psychiatric diagnosis. The clinical implications of this distinction will be discussed in a later section.

Somatization as a Tendency to Seek Care for Common Symptoms

A third model considers the role of psychological distress in determining whether patients seek health care for preexisting symptoms (Figure 3-3). Such a model proposes that unpleasant physical symptoms are ubiquitous and that negative affective states cause people to seek health care for symptoms they might otherwise ignore. Mechanic (1972) has argued that psychological distress causes somatizing patients to interpret common bodily sensations as evidence of disease. Consequently, emotionally distressed patients visit physicians for common symptoms that others manage without medical attention. Population surveys find that most healthy people frequently experience various mild symptoms for which they do not seek medical care (Reidenberg and Lowenthal 1968). Mechanic's analyses of survey data demonstrate the relationship between psychological distress and health perceptions (Tessler and Mechanic

1978). His longitudinal studies suggest a learned pattern of coping with emotional distress by focusing on bodily symptoms and seeking health care (Mechanic 1979).

Studies of some common somatization syndromes support the hypothesis that psychological factors contribute to somatization by influencing health care decisions. Drossman and colleagues (1988) studied psychiatric morbidity in patients seen in a gastroenterology clinic for symptoms of irritable bowel syndrome (IBS) and compared those subjects to two control groups: community control subjects reporting IBS symptoms but not seeking medical care, and asymptomatic community control subjects. While patients with IBS reported higher levels of psychiatric symptoms, nonpatients with symptoms of this syndrome were not significantly more psychologically distressed than asymptomatic control subjects. Psychiatric morbidity, therefore, was associated with seeking care for irritable bowel symptoms instead of with the symptoms themselves. Whitehead and coworkers (1988) reported similar findings in a comparison of IBS clinic patients with nonpatients reporting similar bowel symptoms. A

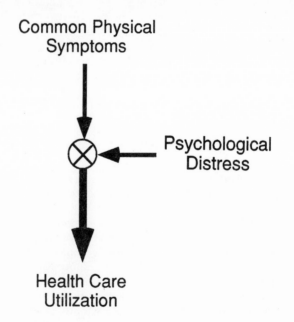

Figure 3-3. Somatization as a tendency to seek care for common symptoms.

similar study of premenstrual syndrome in patients and nonpatients found psychiatric morbidity to be more strongly linked to the decision to seek medical care for menstrual symptoms than to the presence of the symptoms themselves (Lipscomb 1990). These findings suggest that many people experience such menstrual or gastrointestinal symptoms, but those who seek care for such symptoms tend to be psychologically distressed.

Somatization as a Consequence of Health Care Utilization

The fourth model of the interaction of somatization, psychiatric disorders, and health care utilization considers use of health services to be a cause of symptom reporting rather than a consequence (Figure 3-4). This hypothesis emphasizes the tendency of cultural forces and medical providers to reinforce illness behavior and symptom reporting. The medical care system and other social institutions that selectively attend to physical symptoms may contribute to iatrogenic somatization. Mayou (1976) discusses the influence of the medical care system on whether nonspecific distress is expressed through

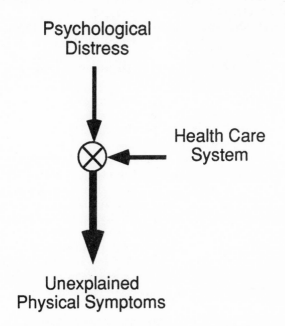

Psychological Distress

Health Care System

Unexplained Physical Symptoms

Figure 3-4. Somatization as a response to the incentives of the health care system.

bodily symptoms. Mechanic (1972) uses the example of frequent somatization among medical students to illustrate how exposure to the medical care system can increase reporting of physical distress.

VALIDATION OF PSYCHIATRIC DIAGNOSES AMONG SOMATIZING PATIENTS

These four models of the process of somatization propose varying roles for psychiatric disorder in the genesis of unexplained physical symptoms. While the traditional model views somatization as an atypical presentation of psychiatric disorder, the other models place less emphasis on specific psychiatric diagnosis. The amplification model raises questions about the validity of traditional psychiatric diagnoses in patients who tend to overreport symptoms in general. Much of the difference between these hypotheses involves uncertainty about the diagnostic meaning of psychiatric symptoms in somatizing patients. This uncertainty about whether reported psychiatric symptoms in somatizing patients indicate discrete psychiatric diagnoses or nonspecific psychological distress raises important clinical questions as well. Resolving these questions would require study of the prevalence of psychiatric disorders in somatizing patients using some other source of information besides self-reported symptoms. Various types of data seem potentially useful, as discussed below.

Biologic Markers of Psychiatric Disorders Among Somatizing Patients

Study of proposed biologic markers of psychiatric illness might provide some validation of psychiatric diagnoses in somatizing patients that is not dependent on self-reported symptoms. Use of such techniques in the somatizing population, however, remains limited. Taerk et al. (1987) reported using a structured psychiatric interview (the DIS), the Beck Depression Inventory, and the dexamethasone suppression test (DST) to examine 24 patients with unexplained postviral fatigue. While two-thirds of the patients had lifetime histories of major depression and almost half had Beck scores showing current depression of at least moderate severity, only one patient showed dexamethasone nonsuppression. Hudson et al. (1984) found dexamethasone nonsuppression in only one of 23 patients with fibromyalgia. Even if more extensive data on dexamethasone suppression among somatizing patients were available, they would likely have little bearing on the validity of depressive diagnoses among somatizing individuals. The DST appears less sensitive to "neurotic" or nonmelancholic depression (Rabkin et al. 1983), and most somatizing patients with apparent depression would fall into this group. Use of sleep EEGs to measure latency until the first REM sleep period has been reported to outperform the DST as a biologic marker of depression (Akiskal et al. 1982). Unfortunately this technique has not been applied to the study of somatization. Among psychiatric disorders for which a heritable component has been demonstrated, family history of disorder suggests a biological disease predisposition. An increased prevalence of typical major depression (not complicated by somatization) among the relatives of somatizing patients would argue for a biological association between somatization and depression. Overall, existing data on biologic markers of psychiatric disorder in somatizing patients yield no clear conclusions, and available techniques have limited potential.

Response of Somatization to Psychiatric Treatment

Response to specific treatment for depression might be considered another external validation of depressive diagnoses in somatizing patients. Existing data on response to antidepressant treatment among these patients remain sketchy. Two controlled studies (Carette et al. 1986; Goldenberg et al. 1986) of low dose amitriptyline in fibromyalgia reported significant benefit. Wysenberk and colleagues (1985), however, reported no benefit among 23 fibromyalgia patients treated with low-dose imipramine in an open trial. Schulberg et al. (1987) studied the clinical course of depression presenting in primary-care medical clinics and found little relation between antidepressant treatment and clinical improvement. The sample, however, was not limited to somatizing patients, and the number of cases was quite small. Even if more relevant data were available, response to antidepressants could provide only limited evidence for or against the validity of psychiatric diagnoses in somatizing patients. Because of the wide range of psychiatric and other diagnoses that respond to tricyclic antidepressants, a positive response among somatizing patients would not necessarily imply the presence of major depression. The various central and peripheral effects of tricyclics might affect functional somatic symptoms through some other mechanism besides the treatment of depression (e.g., anticholinergic effects on irritable bowel complaints). Further, because of the significant proportion of patients with typical major depression who fail to improve with tricyclic treatment, a low response rate in somatizing patients would not prove the absence of depressive illness.

Validation of Psychiatric Diagnoses Using Symptom Patterns

Analysis of the patterns of psychiatric-symptom reporting among somatizing patients could provide another method for examining the validity of psychiatric diagnoses. If psychiatric symptoms in somatizing patients truly indicate underlying psychiatric diagnoses, then the patterns of psychiatric-symptom reporting among these patients should resemble those in nonsomatizing patients with typical psychiatric disorders. If psychiatric symptoms among somatizing patients result instead from a nonspecific tendency to overreport distress, the pattern of symptom reporting should reveal no underlying pattern except generalized symptom amplification. Blazer et al. (1988) applied grade-of-membership analysis, a new technique for examining the underlying structure of diagnostic information, to the study of psychiatric symptoms among medical-service users. In that group the structure of symptom reports closely resembled established psychiatric diagnoses. Use of similar methods to study psychiatric symptoms among somatizing patients might help determine whether those symptoms indicate specific diagnoses or nonspecific amplification.

IMPLICATIONS FOR CLINICAL CARE

Each of the four models of somatization discussed above has practical implications for the clinical care of somatizing patients. Although the various models are presented as if mutually exclusive, each of these processes probably makes some contribution in every case. The prudent psychiatric or primary care clinician will look to each theory for whatever useful intervention it might contribute. Our current treatment of somatization is not so effective that we can afford to overlook any potentially helpful strategy.

The first model focuses on treatment of the conventional psychiatric disorder presumed to lie beneath unexplained physical symptoms. Because unexplained physical symptoms are presumed to be "masked" expressions of depression and anxiety, conventional pharmacological and psychotherapeutic treatment of these disorders should relieve the accompanying physical symptoms.

One unfortunate consequence of the focus on "masked" psychiatric disorders is that patients sometimes feel profoundly misunderstood. Although many patients with unexplained physical symptoms will report depression and anxiety, they invariably view these psychiatric symptoms as consequences of physical symptoms instead of causes. When told that their physical discomfort results from depression or anxiety, such patients typically respond with anger and disbelief. Often patients feel that assignment of a psychiatric diagnosis dismisses distressing physical symptoms as being "all in your head." A traditional view of somatization would explain this reaction as defense and resistance. Somatizing patients' distressed protests would be seen as confirmation of their underlying depression or anxiety, and of their need to defend against it.

Reports of the difficulties encountered during treatment of somatizing patients illustrate the limitation of a traditional approach. Roberts (1977) and Ford and Long (1977) both describe their experience with psychodynamically oriented group treatment of somatization. Both accounts describe somatizing patients as psychologically defended and resistant to psychological insight. Patients frequently responded to interpretive efforts with avoidance and discontinuation of treatment.

Treatment based on the amplification model of somatization focuses on strategies to reduce underlying symptom sensitivity. Somatosensory amplification is viewed as a perceptual style amenable to change through cognitive and behavioral interventions. Barsky and colleagues (1988a) have described a group treatment program with a psychoeducational and supportive orientation. Distraction and relaxation techniques assist patients to reduce sensitivity to bodily sensations. Cognitive interventions allow somatizing patients to reattribute physical sensations to benign causes. Supportive discussions of life stresses and situational factors help to relieve the overall psychological distress driving the amplification process. The entire process considers patients' physical symptoms genuine expressions of distress deserving of attention. Physical distress is not a defense against the real problem; it is the real problem. This focus on symptom reduction helps to build a collaborative relationship based on attempts at palliation.

The third model of somatization views psychological distress as the catalyst that motivates patients to seek medical care for preexisting physical symptoms. One important consequence of this model is its reminder to us that vague physical symptoms may have causes independent of the psychological distress that induce patients to visit doctors. A patient with chest pain whose current clinic visit is motivated by emotional distress may still have ischemic heart disease. All of the preceding discussion of somatization should not be considered an argument that emotionally distressed patients are immune to medical illnesses. This model, however, encourages us to focus on two aspects of the patient's presentation. We should consider first what process might be causing the current symptoms. This exploration begins with the basics of medical diagnosis. We then should consider why this patient has sought care for these symptoms at this time. The important contribution of this theoretical model is that the causes of the patient's current illness and the reasons for seeking care may be completely independent of each other. Just as the presence of emotional distress does not preclude an underlying medical disorder, the presence of a definitive medical diagnosis does not entirely explain what made a particular patient choose to visit a doctor. Effective treatment must consider both sides of any clinical presentation.

The fourth model of somatization discussed above emphasizes the role of the medical care system in fostering symptom reporting and illness behavior. Treatment strategies based on this model attempt to minimize the rewards associated with the patient role. Physicians caring for somatizing patients are encouraged not to make care and attention dependent on continued illness and disability. Somatizing patients should receive regular appointments not contingent on the development of new symptoms or on old ones becoming worse. Providers thus emphasize that patients need not become or remain sick in order to maintain the doctor-patient relationship. Focusing treatment on symptomatic relief instead of diagnostic exploration reduces the incentive to present more symptoms in order to receive more diagnostic tests. Providers should view emotional symptoms as genuine problems deserving as much care and attention as physical ones. Such an approach reduces patients' incentives to present distress through bodily symptoms.

In this chapter I have considered various explanations for the strong interrelationships among unexplained physical symptoms, psychiatric symptoms, and use of health services. The various theories discussed view somatization as an intrapsychic defense, a manifestation of aberrant neurobiology, a system of perception and cognition, and a set of social behaviors. Available evidence supports the importance of each of these views. In this way our understanding of the process of somatization mirrors our understanding of other psychiatric syndromes. Many theoretical orientations inform our clinical practice, and we serve our patients best by remaining open to help from any theoretical direction.

REFERENCES

Akiskal HS, Lemmi H, Yerevanian B: The utility of the REM latency test in psychiatric diagnosis: a study of 81 depressed outpatients. Psychiatry Res 7:101–110, 1982

American Psychiatric Association: Diagnostic and Statistical Manual of Mental Disorders, 3rd Edition. Washington, DC, American Psychiatric Association, 1980

American Psychiatric Association: Diagnostic and Statistical Manual of Mental Disorders, 3rd Edition, Revised. Washington, DC, American Psychiatric Association, 1987

Balint M: The Doctor, His Patient, and the Illness. New York, International Universities Press, 1957

Barrett JE, Barrett JA, Oxman TE, et al: The prevalence of psychiatric disorders in a primary care practice. Arch Gen Psychiatry 45:1100–1106, 1988

Barsky AJ: Patients who amplify bodily sensations. Ann Intern Med 91:63–70, 1979

Barsky AJ, Klerman GL: Overview: hypochondriasis, bodily complaints, and somatic styles. Am J Psychiatry 140:273–283, 1983

Barsky AJ, Geringer E, Wool CA: A cognitive-educational treatment for hypochondriasis. Gen Hosp Psychiatry 10:322–327, 1988a

Barsky AJ, Goodson JD, Lane RS, et al: The amplification of somatic symptoms. Psychosom Med 50:510–519, 1988b

Blazer D, Swartz M, Woodbury M, et al: Depressive symptoms and depressive diagnoses in a community population: use of a new procedure for analysis of psychiatric classification. Arch Gen Psychiatry 45:1078–1084, 1988

Bohman M, Cloninger CR, von Knorring A, et al: A study of somatoform disorders: cross fostering analysis and genetic relationship to alcoholism and criminality. Arch Gen Psychiatry 41:872–878, 1984

Buschbaum MS: Average evoked response and stimulus intensity in identical and fraternal twins. Physiological Psychology 2:365–370, 1974

Buschbaum MS, Silverman J: Stimulus intensity control and the cortical evoked response. Psychosom Med 30:12–22, 1968

Byrne D: Repression-sensitization as a dimension of personality, in Progress in Experimental Personality Research. Edited by Maher BA. New York, Academic, 1964, pp 169–220

Byrne D, Steinberg MA, Schwartz MS: Relationship between repression-sensitization and physical illness. J Abnorm Psychol 73:154–155, 1968

Carette S, McCain GA, Bell DA, et al: Evaluation of amitriptyline in primary fibrositis. Arthritis Rheum 29:655–659, 1986

Clancy J, Noyes R: Anxiety neurosis: a disease for the medical model. Psychosomatics 17:90–93, 1976

Cormier LE, Katon W, Russo J, et al: Chest pain with negative cardiac diagnostic studies: relationship to psychiatric illness. J Nerv Ment Dis 176:351–358, 1988

Costa PT, McCrae RR: Somatic complaints in males as a function of age and neuroticism: a longitudinal analysis. J Behav Med 3:245–255, 1980

Costa PT, McCrae RR: Hypochondriasis, neuroticism, and aging: when are somatic complaints unfounded? Am Psychol 40:19–28, 1985

Derogatis LR, Lipman RS, Covi L: SCL-90: an outpatient psychiatric rating scale: preliminary report. Psychopharmacol Bull 9:13–27, 1973

Drossman DA, McKee DC, Sandler RS, et al: Psychosocial factors in the irritable bowel syndrome. Gastroenterology 95:701–708, 1988

Escobar JI, Burnam A, Karno M, et al: Somatization in the community. Arch Gen Psychiatry 44:713–718, 1987a

Escobar JI, Golding JM, Hough RL, et al: Somatization in the community: relationship to disability and use of services. Am J Public Health 77:837–840, 1987b

Flor-Henry P, Fromm-Auch D, Tapper M, et al: A neuropsychological study of the stable syndrome of hysteria. Biol Psychiatry 16:601–626, 1981

Ford CV, Long KD: Group therapy of somatizing patients. Psychother Psychosom 28:294–304, 1977

Fossey MD, Lydiard RB, Marsh WH, et al: Prevalence of psychiatric morbidity in irritable bowel syndrome. Paper presented at the annual meeting of the American Psychiatric Association, San Francisco, CA, May 1989

Goldenberg DL: Psychiatric and psychologic aspects of the fibromyalgia syndrome. Rheum Dis Clin North Am 15:105–114, 1989

Goldenberg DL, Felson DT, Dinerman H: A randomized, controlled trial of amitriptyline and naproxen in the treatment of patients with fibrositis. Arthritis Rheum 29:1371–1377, 1986

Hanback JW, Revelle W: Arousal and perceptual sensitivity in hypochondriacs. J Abnorm Psychol 37:523–530, 1978

Hankin JR, Locke BZ: The persistence of depressive symptomatology among prepaid group practice enrollees: an exploratory study. Am J Public Health 72:1000–1007, 1982

Hudson JI, Pliner LF, Hudson MS, et al: The dexamethasone suppression test in fibrositis. Biol Psychiatry 19:1489–1493, 1984

Hudson JI, Hudson MS, Pliner LF, et al: Fibromyalgia and major affective disorder: a controlled phenomenology and family history study. Am J Psychiatry 142:441–446, 1985

Imboden JB, Canter A, Cluff LE: Convalescence from influenza. Arch Intern Med 108:115–121, 1961

Jackson D: In the library. Chronic Fatigue and Immune Dysfunction Syndrome Association Chronicle, Nov/Dec 1988, pp 31–35

Jones LR, Badger LW, Ficken RP, et al: Inside the hidden mental health network: examining the mental health care delivery of primary care physicians. Gen Hosp Psychiatry 9:287–293, 1987

Kaplan C, Lipkin M, Gordon GH: Somatization in primary care: patients with unexplained and vexing medical complaints. J Gen Intern Med 3:177–190, 1988

Katon W, Kleinman A, Rosen G: Depression and somatization: a review. Am J Med 72:127–135, 241–247, 1982

Kellner R: Functional somatic symptoms and hypochondriasis. Arch Gen Psychiatry 42:821–833, 1985

Kessler LG, Cleary PD, Burke JD Jr: Psychiatric disorders in primary care: results of a follow-up study. Arch Gen Psychiatry 42:583–587, 1985

Kessler LG, Burns BJ, Shapiro S, et al: Psychiatric diagnoses of medical service users: evidence from the Epidemiologic Catchment Area program. Am J Public Health 77:18–24, 1987

Lipscomb P: Psychiatric correlates of medical utilization in women with premenstrual syndrome. Journal of Psychosomatic Obstetrics and Gynecology 2:129, 1990

Martin RL, Roberts WV, Clayton PJ, et al: Psychiatric illness and non-cancer hysterectomy. Diseases of the Nervous System 38:974–980, 1977

Mathew RJ, Weinman ML, Mirabi M: Physical symptoms of depression. Br J Psychiatry 139:293–296, 1981

Mayou R: The nature of bodily symptoms. Br J Psychiatry 129:55–60, 1976

Meares R, Horvath T: "Acute" and "chronic" hysteria. Br J Psychiatry 121:653–657, 1972

Mechanic D: Social psychologic factors affecting the presentation of bodily complaints. N Engl J Med 286:1132–1139, 1972

Mechanic D: Development of psychological distress among young adults. Arch Gen Psychiatry 36:1233–1239, 1979

Miller LA: Neuropsychological concepts of somatoform disorders. Int J Psychiatry Med 14:31–46, 1984

Myalgic Encephalomyelitis Society: M.E. and You. Auckland, New Zealand, Myalgic Encephalomyelitis Society, 1985

Nemiah JC: Alexithymia. Psychother Psychosom 28:199–206, 1977

Nielsen AC, Williams TA: Depression in ambulatory medical patients. Arch Gen Psychiatry 37:999–1004, 1980

Oxman TE, Rosenberg SD, Schnurr PP, et al: Linguistic dimensions of affect and thought in somatization disorder. Am J Psychiatry 142:1150–1155, 1985

Pennebaker JW: The Psychology of Physical Symptoms. New York, Springer-Verlag, 1982

Pennebaker JW, Burnam MA, Schaeffer MA, et al: Lack of control as a determinant of perceived physical symptoms. J Pers Soc Psychol 35:167–174, 1977

Petrie A: Individuality in Pain and Suffering, 2nd Edition. Chicago, IL, University of Chicago Press, 1978

Rabkin JG, Quitkin FM, Stewart JW, et al: The dexamethasone suppression test with mildly to moderately depressed outpatients. Am J Psychiatry 140:926–927, 1983

Raine AR, Mitchell DA, Venables PH: Cortical augmenting-reducing: modality specific? Psychophysiology 18:700–708, 1981

Regier DA, Boyd JH, Burke JD, et al: One-month prevalence of mental disorders in the United States: based on five Epidemiologic Catchment Area sites. Arch Gen Psychiatry 45:977–986, 1988

Reidenberg MM, Lowenthal DT: Adverse nondrug reactions. N Engl J Med 279:678–679, 1968

Roberts JP: The problems of group psychotherapy for psychosomatic patients. Psychother Psychosom 28:305–315, 1977

Schulberg HC, McClelland M, Gooding W: Six-month outcomes for medical patients with major depressive disorders. J Gen Intern Med 2:312–317, 1987

Schurman RA, Kramer PD, Mitchell JB: The hidden mental health network. Arch Gen Psychiatry 42:89–94, 1985

Sherry S, Notman M, Nadelson CC, et al: Anxiety, depression, and menstrual symptoms among freshman medical students. J Clin Psychiatry 49:490–493, 1988

Silver H: Physical complaints are part of the core depressive syndrome: evidence from a cross-cultural study in Israel. J Clin Psychiatry 48:140–142, 1987

Simon GE: Physical symptoms of psychiatric disorder. Psychosom Med 52:224, 1990

Simon GE, Katon WJ, Sparks PJ: Allergic to life: psychologic factors in environmental illness. Am J Psychiatry 147:901–908, 1990

Smith GR, Monson RA, Ray DC: Patients with multiple unexplained symptoms: their characteristics, functional health, and health care utilization. Arch Intern Med 146:69–72, 1986

Stewart MA, McWhinney IR, Buck CW: How illness presents: a study of patient behavior. J Fam Pract 2:411–414, 1975

Sullivan MD, Katon W, Dobie R, et al: Disabling tinnitus: association with affective disorder. Gen Hosp Psychiatry 10:285–291, 1988

Swartz M, Hughes D, Blazer D, et al: Somatization disorder in the community: a study of diagnostic concordance among three diagnostic systems. J Nerv Ment Dis 175:26–33, 1987

Taerk GS, Toner BB, Salit IE, et al: Depression in patients with neuromyasthenia (benign myalgic encephalitis). Int J Psychiatry Med 17:49–56, 1987

Tessler R, Mechanic D: Psychologic distress and perceived health status. J Health Soc Behav 19:254–262, 1978

Torgerson S: Genetics of somatoform disorders. Arch Gen Psychiatry 43:502–505, 1986

von Knorring L, Perris C: Biochemistry of the augmenting-reducing response in visual evoked potentials. Neuropsychobiology 7:1–8, 1981

Von Korff M, Shapiro S, Burke JD, et al: Anxiety and depression in a primary care clinic: comparison of Diagnostic Interview Schedule, General Health Questionnaire, and practitioner assessments. Arch Gen Psychiatry 44:152–156, 1987

Walker E, Katon W, Harrop-Griffiths J, et al: Relationship of chronic pelvic pain to psychiatric diagnoses and childhood sexual abuse. Am J Psychiatry 145:75–80, 1988

Watson D, Clark LA: Negative affectivity: the disposition to experience aversive emotional states. Psychol Bull 96:465–490, 1984

Watson D, Tellegen A: Toward a consensual model of mood. Psychol Bull 98:219–235, 1985

Waxman HM, McReary G, Weinrit RM, et al: A comparison of somatic complaints among depressed and non-depressed older persons. Gerontologist 25:501–507, 1985

Whitehead WE, Bosmajian L, Zonderman AB, et al: Symptoms of psychologic distress associated with irritable bowel syndrome. Gastroenterology 95:709–714, 1988

Williams P, Tarnopolsky A, Hand D, et al: Minor psychiatric morbidity and general practice consultations: the West London Survey. Psychol Med 9 (suppl):1–37, 1986

Wysenberk AJ, Mor F, Lurie Y, et al: Imipramine for the treatment of fibrositis: a therapeutic trial. Ann Rheum Dis 44:752–753, 1985

Young SJ, Alpers DH, Norland CC, et al: Psychiatric illness and the irritable bowel syndrome: practical implications for the primary care physician. Gastroenterology 70:162–166, 1976

Zoccolillo MS, Cloninger R: Excess medical care of women with somatization disorder. South Med J 79:532–535, 1986

Chapter 4

Medically Unexplained Symptoms: Distribution, Risk Factors, and Comorbidity

Javier I. Escobar, M.D., Marvin Swartz, M.D.,
Maritza Rubio-Stipec, M.A., Peter Manu, M.D.

P roper assessment of patients presenting with medically unexplained symptoms is often delayed by a lack of effective collaboration between medical and mental-health specialists as a result of their limited and differing perspectives. Indeed, current psychiatric terms and nosologies for these symptomatic presentations remain absent from recent editions of leading medical and neurological textbooks. In those sources, "hysteria," "hypochondriasis," and "malingering" are still used when referring to patients with unexplained symptoms (Escobar et al. 1989).

A psychogenic etiology for medically unexplained symptoms is largely inferred from the association of symptoms with specific "stressors," putative psychological gain, coexistence of somatic symptoms and symptoms of another psychiatric disorder, or a psychogenic diagnosis of exclusion ("If it is not physical, it has to be psychological"). The guiding principle is that the medically unexplained symptom represents a somatic idiom for the expression of psychological distress. Obviously, this is a matter of clinical inference, and, lacking reliable or measurable parameters, the ascription of psychiatric causes to symptoms may often be arbitrary. We therefore feel it would be preferable to use the more generic phrase "medically unexplained physical symptoms" in lieu of terms such as "somatization" or "somatoform symptoms" as a unifying nosological theme at this stage of our knowledge.

In the pre-DSM-III era the concepts of somatization, hypochon-

---

This chapter is a revised version of a paper presented at the 142nd annual meeting of the American Psychiatric Association, San Francisco, California, May 8, 1989.

driasis, and hysteria were used to indicate possible psychiatric etiologies (Barsky and Klerman 1983). Although often used pejoratively, these concepts seemed to provide a consensual characterization of many patients. The furor for purely descriptive categories in DSM-III changed both the denotation and the connotation of these terms. Thus, the term "somatization" was borrowed to rename a well-validated and operationally defined syndrome (hysteria/ Briquet's syndrome), "hysteria" was renamed "conversion," and "hypochondriasis" was kept relatively intact. The goal in DSM-III of creating discrete somatoform entities was only partially successful. With the exception of somatization disorder, the discriminant validity of other somatoform disorders remains unproven (Bishop and Torch 1979; Hyler and Sussman 1984).

In the introductory chapter of this book, Kirmayer and Robbins select the term "somatization" to encompass those somatic manifestations with a psychiatric etiology. Besides providing a useful review of the somatization concept, the authors outline three relatively discrete forms of somatization:

1. High levels (numbers) of medically unexplained symptoms. (This form includes DSM-III-R somatization disorder and other subsyndromal somatization constructs.)
2. Amplifying somatic styles (similar to DSM-III-R's hypochondriasis).
3. Somatic presentations associated with a primary psychiatric disorder (e.g., chest pain and panic disorder, muscle weakness, pain complaints, and major depressive disorder).

In this chapter we describe an operational construct that may capture at least partially some of the above subtypes and may prove to be of practical value in medical settings as a rather nonintrusive tool to screen for somatization disorder and other types of psychopathology (Manu et al. 1989, in press).

IS THERE A NATURAL AGGREGATION OF SOMATIC SYMPTOMS?

Because the original somatization disorder criteria (that of hysteria/Briquet's syndrome) were based on clinical studies of polysymptomatic individuals, it seemed prudent to take advantage of large epidemiologic surveys recently completed and explore whether or not there was a natural aggregation of such symptoms without making a priori assumptions. Using a large community population

Swartz et al. (1986a) explored the "natural" clustering of somatic symptoms using a multivariate technique (grade-of-membership [or GOM] analysis) in analyses that included all the DSM-III somatic items as elicited with the Diagnostic Interview Schedule (DIS) (Robins et al. 1981). The DIS elicits 37 possible symptoms to diagnose DSM-III somatization disorder. These symptoms relate to common manifestations of the gastrointestinal, cardiopulmonary, genitourinary, neurological, and musculoskeletal systems and include most of those symptoms often related to psychological or emotional factors (e.g., lump in throat, paralysis, aphonia, palpitations, dizziness). To meet DIS/DSM-III criteria, the symptom must reach a severity threshold (interfere with function, lead to physician visits, and/or lead to prescription medication intake) and should not be explainable by physical illness or injury, or by the use of medications, drugs, or alcohol.

The GOM analyses yielded several somatic-symptom clusters. Table 4-1 lists the three major types (IV, V, and VII). Note from the table that one of these clusters (type V) closely resembles the polysymptomatic categories of hysteria/Briquet's syndrome and DSM-III somatization disorder both in symptom profile and in demographic characteristics. Two other clusters (types IV and VII) that included fewer symptoms were found predominantly among male respondents. The symptoms in type IV were primarily pain and conversion symptoms somewhat resembling DSM-III-R somatoform pain disorder, while those in type VII were mainly cardiorespiratory. These data support the validity of the Briquet's syndrome–somatization disorder concept. However, they call into question the separation of symptom-based somatoform disorders into the many current DSM-III-R categories. Assuming a dimensional rather than a categorical model of somatoform phenomena, it is conceivable that some of the remaining DSM-III-R categories (except perhaps hypochondriasis) could be lumped into similar clusters of medically unexplained symptoms.

In Puerto Rico, Rubio-Stipec et al. (1989), also using multivariate techniques in analyses that included the full range of DIS and DSM-III symptoms and diagnoses, identified five symptom scales with high internal consistency. One scale consisted of a somatic-symptoms factor. (The other scales were "affective," "anxiety," "psychosis," and "alcohol.") Interestingly, similar factor analyses performed with the St. Louis Epidemiologic Catchment Area (ECA) and the Los Angeles ECA data sets failed to isolate a somatic-symptoms factor while replicating the other four factors, suggesting that the somatic-symptoms factor may be unique to Puerto Rican

Table 4-1.   Diagnostic Interview Schedule somatic symptom
clusters found in two community surveys

Puerto Rico's somatic factor[a]	Durham's GOM clusters[b]		
	Type IV	Type V	Type VII
Gastrointestinal symptoms			
Abdominal pain	–None–	Abdominal pain	–None–
Nausea		Nausea	
Vomiting		Vomiting	
Excessive gas		Excessive gas	
		Diarrhea	
		Constipation	
		Food intolerance	
Cardiorespiratory symptoms			
Dyspnea	Dyspnea	–None–	Dyspnea
Chest pain			Chest pain
Palpitations			Palpitations
Pseudoneurological symptoms			
Unusual spells	Trouble walking	Unusual spells	Fainting
Amnesia	Lump in throat	Amnesia	Dizziness
Paralysis	Lost voice	Seizures	Blurred vision
Dizziness		Deafness	
Fainting		Blindness	
Musculoskeletal symptoms			
–None–	Back pain	–None–	–None–
	Joint pain		
	Extremity pain		
Other pain			
–None–	–None–	Headache	Headache
		Mouth pain	
Genitourinary symptoms			
–None–	–None–	Pain (urination)	–None–
		Pain (genitals)	
		Pain (intercourse)	
		Sex unpleasurable	
Miscellaneous symptoms			
Sickly	Muscle weakness	Sickly	–None–
Muscle weakness			

Note.   GOM = grade-of-membership (see text).
[a]From Rubio-Stipec et al. 1989.
[b]From Swartz et al. 1986a.

populations (Rubio-Stipec et al. 1989). Interestingly, this factor appears to be a blend of Swartz et al.'s clusters V and VII.

AN ABRIDGED SOMATIZATION CONSTRUCT

Prevalence of DSM-III Somatization Disorder and the Need for an Abridged Construct

Using DSM-III criteria, community studies with the DIS showed that the prevalence of somatization disorder at six epidemiologic sites ranged between 0 and 0.7% and averaged about 0.1% (see Table 4-2).

Since somatization disorder was the only DSM-III somatoform diagnosis included in the DIS, and in view of its low observed prevalence, one of the present authors (J.I.E.) began exploring below-threshold counts of somatization disorder symptoms elicited with the DIS in efforts to develop the construct of an abridged or sub-syndromal somatization disorder. The idea was to capture a significant portion of those individuals traditionally labeled as "somatizers" or "hypochondriacs" prior to DSM-III who, in spite of presenting various somatic symptoms and concerns, would not meet criteria for full somatization disorder. The development of such an abridged construct assumed that, rather than being discrete entities, the various somatoform syndromes may lie on a somatoform continuum. In this dimensional model, somatization disorder would be placed at the "severe" extreme, while other syndromes such as hypochondriasis, somatoform pain disorder, undifferentiated and atypical somatoform disorders, and the somatic manifestations coexisting with affective and anxiety syndromes would represent less severe or evolving forms of

Table 4-2. Lifetime prevalence of an abridged somatization construct (SSI 4,6) and somatization disorder at five United States sites and the island of Puerto Rico

Site	SSI 4,6 (%)	SD (%)
Baltimore	9	0.1
Durham	20	0.4
Los Angeles	9	0.0
New Haven	N/A	0.2
St. Louis	10	0.1
Puerto Rico	20	0.7

Note. SSI = Somatic Symptoms Index. SD = somatization disorder.
Source. Modified from Swartz et al., in press, and Escobar et al. 1989.

somatization disorder. (For example, with the passage of time, more lifetime symptoms would accrue until the somatization disorder threshold would eventually be reached.) The abridged construct was developed and validated in studies using the DIS (Escobar et al. 1987a, 1987b, 1989). This construct requires the presence (lifetime) of at least four medically unexplained physical symptoms for males and six for females from the 37 criterion symptoms included in the DIS somatization disorder section. The community prevalence of this abridged construct, presented in Table 4-2, was 50 to 100 times greater than that reported for somatization disorder.

The abridged construct has also been referred to as "somatization syndrome" (Swartz et al., in press). Because it is basically a somatic-symptoms count, the use of the more descriptive term *Somatic Symptom Index 4,6* (SSI 4,6) has recently been proposed (Escobar et al. 1989). (The digits refer to the number of symptoms necessary to reach criterion level for male and female subjects, respectively.) In this notation, DSM-III somatization disorder can be abbreviated as SSI 14,16, DSM III-R somatization disorder as SSI 13, and so forth.

Testing the Abridged Somatization Construct

The abridged somatization cutoffs were initially tested on a sample of more than 3,000 community respondents in Los Angeles as part of the Epidemiologic Catchment Area (ECA) Project (Escobar et al. 1987a; Karno et al. 1987). A majority of the respondents represented two large ethnic groups (Mexican Americans and non-Hispanic whites). The data showed that while the prevalence of "full" DSM-III somatization disorder was only 0.03%, that of the abridged construct (SSI 4,6) was over 100 times greater (Escobar et al. 1987a). Sociodemographic and psychopathological correlates were associated with abridged somatization (SSI 4,6) in the expected direction. Thus, advancing age, female gender, and the presence of a psychiatric diagnosis (particularly major depression or dysthymia) were positively related to increased somatization. Ethnic differences could be documented only for females, and Mexican-American women had a greater prevalence of SSI 4,6 than did their non-Hispanic white counterparts (Escobar et al. 1987a).

The SSI 4,6 construct was then tested in two other large epidemiologic samples—the full ECA and the Puerto Rican epidemiologic samples—that used very similar methodologies employing the DIS to interview probability samples of community respondents. In addition to the Los Angeles sample, the full ECA sample included respondents from Baltimore, Durham (N.C.), New Haven, and St. Louis, for a total of almost 20,000 respondents

(Swartz et al., in press). In Puerto Rico the data included over 1,500 community respondents interviewed in an island-wide survey (Canino et al. 1987). The data (see Table 4-2) indicate that prevalences of full and abridged somatization were higher in Puerto Rico and Durham than at the other sites. The differences between Durham and the other United States ECA sites may result from the large sample of rural blacks interviewed in Durham, since, as can be seen in Table 4-3, black respondents reported high prevalences of medically unexplained symptoms, somatization disorder, and abridged somatization (Swartz et al., in press). The fact that investigators in both Durham and Puerto Rico applied a more stringent "medical editing" of somatic item responses than did investigators at the other sites may also account for some of these differences. Such medical editing tends to lead to more symptoms being scored as unexplained on the DIS because many explanations offered by respondents are rejected by the reviewing physician as implausible. However, analyses with the "unedited" Puerto Rican data compared with the Los Angeles data still revealed significant differences between the two samples (Escobar et al. 1989).

Regarding ethnic distribution, Puerto Ricans had the highest rates of full and abridged somatization, followed by North American blacks, while United States Hispanics (who were largely of Mexican-American descent) showed overall rates similar to those of non-Hispanic whites (Table 4-3). Secondary analyses of the Los Angeles data showed that Mexican-American females, particularly those over the age of 45 years, reported higher somatic-symptoms counts and higher rates of "abridged" somatization than did younger Mexican-American women and their non-Hispanic white counterparts (Escobar et al. 1987a). Many of these differences, however, were erased when the analyses were controlled for educational level (Escobar et al. 1989).

In the United States and Puerto Rico, gender and educational levels

Table 4-3. Ethnic distribution of an abridged somatization construct (SSI 4,6) and somatization disorder

Ethnic group	SSI 4,6 (%)	SD (%)
Blacks (United States)	15	0.4
Non-Hispanic whites (United States)	11	0.1
Hispanics (United States)	11	0.0
Puerto Ricans (Puerto Rico)	20	0.7

Note. SSI = Somatic Symptoms Index. SD = somatization disorder.

were related to both full and abridged somatization, although the effect of gender in Puerto Ricans was seen only in the oldest age group (Tables 4-4 and 4-5). The relationship of somatization and age seems strong only in the case of Puerto Rican respondents.

Table 4-4. Sociodemographic factors (United States Epidemiologic Catchment Area sample only)

Sociodemographic factor	SSI 4,6 (%)	SD (%)
Age		
Below 45 years	11	0.1
45 years and older	11	0.1
Sex		
Male	9	0.0
Female	14	0.2
Education		
High school graduates	10	0.0
Non–high school graduates	15	0.2

Note. SSI = Somatic Symptoms Index. SD = somatization disorder.
Source. Modified from Swartz et al. 1986b.

Table 4-5. Age and sex distribution of an abridged somatization construct (SSI 4,6) in Puerto Rico

	Prevalence of SSI 4,6	
Age group	Males (%)	Females (%)
18–29	14	11
30–39	16	16
40–49	24	23
50 and over	21	33

Note. SSI = Somatic Symptoms Index.
Source. Modified from Escobar et al. 1989.

Somatization in a Medical Sample of Patients With Persistent Fatigue

Manu et al. (1988) have studied over 200 patients who presented with a primary complaint of persistent fatigue at the Department of Internal Medicine, University of Connecticut Health Center in Farmington, Connecticut. Patients underwent a thorough physical and psychiatric assessment that included the DIS administered by an internist (P.M.). Over one-half of the patients (51%) met criteria (lifetime) for abridged somatization (SSI 4,6), while 12.5% met criteria for "full" somatization disorder (SSI 13 [DSM-III-R]). Interestingly, over one-half of the patients ($n = 103$) also met criteria for recent (within 6 months) major depression, and 13% met criteria for recent panic disorder. In only 5% of the 200 cases was a physical disorder identified, after a thorough workup, as a possible cause for the symptoms. In 20% of the patients, the fatigue was not explained by a current physical or psychiatric disorder.

Figure 4-1 depicts the prevalence of somatization disorder and SSI 4,6 in the epidemiologic and clinical populations we have studied thus far with the DIS. Note that, as expected, the medical sample present-

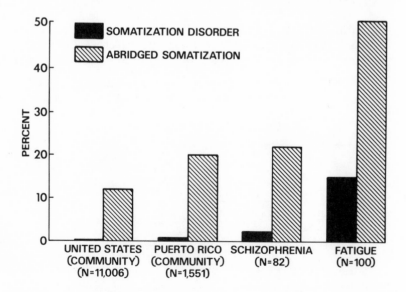

Figure 4-1. Frequency of full and abridged somatization disorder (Somatic Symptom Index 4,6) in four studies.

ing with fatigue constitutes the largest proportion of somatizing individuals, followed by the psychiatric sample and the community sample from Puerto Rico.

Validity of the Abridged Somatization Construct

Psychiatric comorbidity. Figures 4-2 and 4-3 show the DIS and DSM-III disorders that coexist with "abridged" somatization in the fatigue and community samples described in Figure 4-1. Note from the figures the similarity in the comorbidity profiles (except for the "alcohol" diagnoses). Note also that while two-thirds of the individuals meet criteria for some disorder, the remaining one-third or so in either sample do not meet criteria for any other current psychiatric disorders (i.e., "pure" somatizers). As expected, major depression, phobia, dysthymia, and panic were the diagnoses most often observed in individuals with high numbers of medically unexplained physical symptoms.

Use of health and mental health services. One of the distinguishing features of somatization (as a process or disorder) is that it leads to avid use of available health care services and, more strikingly, to a preferential use of medical services over mental health services (Escobar et al. 1987b). The ECA survey scrutinized patterns of service use. Table 4-6 shows the data for the full community sample broken down by somatization status. The data indicate that individuals with somatization disorder show the greatest likelihood of using health care services and that those with abridged somatization (SSI 4,6)

Table 4-6. An abridged somatization construct (SSI 4,6), somatization disorder, and the use of health and mental health services at four Epidemiologic Catchment Area sites

Type of service used (period)	Percent using services		
	SSI 4,6 %	SD %	Neither %
Outpatient (past 6 months)			
General health	77	95	56
Specialty mental health	34	56	8
Inpatient (past year)			
General health	27	45	11
Specialty mental health	2	16	0

Note. SSI = Somatic Symptoms Index. SD = somatization disorder.
Source. Modified from Swartz et al., in press.

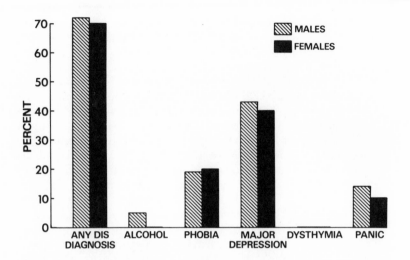

Figure 4-2. Comorbidity of abridged somatization (Somatic Symptoms Index 4,6) (full Epidemiologic Catchment Area sample). DIS = Diagnostic Interview Schedule.

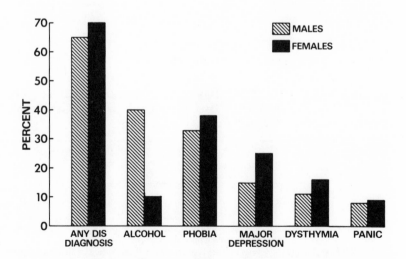

Figure 4-3. Comorbidity of abridged somatization (Somatic Symptoms Index 4,6) (chronic fatigue sample). DIS = Diagnostic Interview Schedule.

follow closely. Table 4-7 uses data from the Los Angeles site and includes only those respondents who, in addition to exceeding the abridged somatization threshold, also met the criteria for at least one other major DIS and DSM-III disorder (except somatization disorder). The data illustrate that SSI 4,6 individuals are more likely to use services than are those below the SSI threshold, and that they also tend to preferentially use medical over mental health services when seeking help for a mental health problem.

Somatization and disability. Community respondents who meet criteria for abridged somatization (SSI 4,6) are more likely than those who do not meet such criteria to report a current disability (Table 4-8). Note that these data are consistent across the different sites

Table 4-7. Use of services by respondents (Los Angeles Epidemiologic Catchment Area sample only) with one or more psychiatric diagnoses who also exceed the threshold for an abridged somatization construct (SSI 4,6)

| | | Percent using service (past year) | | | |
| | | Males | | Females | |
Type of service used	SSI 4,6:	Yes	No	Yes	No
General health		60	2	47	5
Specialty mental health		0	8	25	13

Note. SSI = Somatic Symptoms Index.
Source. Modified from Escobar et al. 1987b.

Table 4-8. An abridged somatization construct (SSI 4,6) and disability (Los Angeles Epidemiologic Catchment Area and Puerto Rico surveys)

| | Percent disabled | |
Site	SSI 4,6 (+)	SSI 4,6 (−)
Los Angeles[a]	58	20
Puerto Rico[b]	15	4

Note. SSI = Somatization Symptoms Index. + indicates respondents who met criteria; − indicates respondents who did not meet criteria.
[a]During the last week respondents report at least 1 day in bed or that physical health interfered significantly with function.
[b]Currently unable to work due to "health problems."
Source. Modified from Escobar and Canino 1989.

(United States and Puerto Rico), although disability was defined differently in the two countries, hence the different percentages. *Somatization and unemployment.* Unemployment was also seen more frequently among somatization disorder and SSI 4,6 respondents. Thus, one-half of the respondents meeting the criteria for somatization disorder, one-third of those meeting the criteria for SSI 4,6, but less than one-fifth of those not meeting the criteria for either construct reported being unemployed 6 months or longer in the past 5 years (Swartz et al., in press).

DISCUSSION

Abridged somatization (SSI 4,6) is a less restrictive cluster of medically unexplained somatic symptoms that can be consistently elicited in clinical and community populations. In a variety of such settings, this construct shows a high prevalence and a consistent association with certain sociodemographic, psychopathological, service-use, disability, and unemployment variables. Unlike full somatization disorder, the abridged construct does not seem to have a gender bias (i.e., prevalences in males and females are similar). Observed patterns in terms of SSI 4,6 distribution and correlates suggest that individuals meeting these criteria may have an abortive or evolving form of somatization disorder. This observation supports a dimensional view of somatization–hypochondriasis phenomena. As currently defined, abridged somatization may incorporate at least major portions of DSM-III-R somatoform disorders (e.g., somatization disorder, hypochondriasis, somatoform pain disorder, and undifferentiated somatoform disorder). One can also visualize in the SSI 4,6 construct major aspects of at least two of the three forms of somatization described by Kirmayer and Robbins in Chapter 1 of this volume (high levels of somatic symptoms and somatic manifestations related to a mood or anxiety disorder).

Indeed, our data indicate that about two-thirds of the respondents who meet the SSI 4,6 criteria also meet the criteria for other (non-somatoform) DSM-III disorders. The remaining third of the SSI 4,6 cohorts (those who do not meet criteria for any other psychiatric disorders) can be viewed as the "pure" somatizing patients and are of particular interest for future study.

The major factors limiting the scope of this research are 1) the "infirmities" of the current instruments, and particularly those affecting the nosologies they aim to elicit, and 2) the problem of comorbidity (because in the comorbid cases it is often very difficult to decide what is "primary," e.g., the somatoform vs. the affective or anxiety syndrome). Also, the reliance of the DIS on lay interviewers without medical knowledge and the possibility of response bias are factors that need to be taken into account for properly interpreting these data. From a more practical perspective, a major limiting factor in the assessment of somatization symptoms is the length of the interview. Thus, each of the 37 symptoms needs to be individually elicited and probed prior to determining specific cutoffs.

To deal with these shortcomings, the use of fewer screening symptoms for somatization disorder has been proposed (Manu et al. 1989; Othmer and De Souza 1985; Smith and Brown 1990; Swartz et al. 1986b). This strategy also looks promising in screening for anxiety and mood disorders in a medical population. Manu et al. (in press) have shown that the number of symptoms to be elicited could be significantly trimmed down from the 37 DSM-III symptoms to the 11 symptoms originally proposed by Swartz et al. (1986). These include five *gastrointestinal* (abdominal pain, nausea, vomiting, diarrhea, flatulence), two *cardiorespiratory* (chest pain, fainting), two *musculoskeletal* (muscle weakness, pain in extremities), and two *miscellaneous* (dizziness, "sickly") symptoms. The presence of five out of these 11 symptoms has been shown to predict somatization disorder in community and medical populations with high levels of sensitivity and specificity (Manu et al. 1989; Swartz et al. 1986b). Also, the use of this index predicted major depression (sensitivity 76%, specificity 88%) and anxiety disorders (sensitivity 96%, specificity 98%) (Manu et al., in press). These findings suggest that the detection of medically unexplained symptoms may have diagnostic value. Eliciting clusters of unexplained physical symptoms may be an unobtrusive way to screen for psychopathology in populations that are not psychologically minded, such as those seen in medical settings. The use of the SSI construct may thus be a good first step in the psychiatric screening of patients presenting with medically unexplained symptoms.

REFERENCES

Barsky AJ, Klerman GL: Overview: hypochondriasis, bodily complaints, and somatic styles. Am J Psychiatry 140:273–283, 1983

Bishop AJ, Torch EM: Dividing hysteria: a preliminary investigation of conversion disorder and psychalgia. J Nerv Ment Dis 167:348–356, 1979

Canino G, Bird HR, Shrout P, et al: The prevalence of specific disorders in Puerto Rico. Arch Gen Psychiatry 44:127–135, 1987

Escobar JI, Canino G: Unexplained physical complaints: psychopathology and epidemiological correlates. Br J Psychiatry 154:24–27, 1989

Escobar JI, Burnam MA, Karno M, et al: Somatization in the community. Arch Gen Psychiatry 44:713–718, 1987a

Escobar JI, Golding JM, Hough RL, et al: Somatization in the community: relationship to disability and use of services. Am J Public Health 77:837–840, 1987b

Escobar JI, Rubio-Stipec M, Canino G, et al: Somatic Symptom Index (SSI): a new and abridged somatization construct: prevalence and epidemiological correlates in two large community samples. J Nerv Ment Dis 177:140–146, 1989

Hyler SE, Sussman N: Somatoform disorders: before and after DSM-III. Hosp Community Psychiatry 35:469–478, 1984

Karno M, Hough RL, Burnam MA, et al: Lifetime prevalence of specific psychiatric disorders among Mexican Americans and non Hispanic whites in Los Angeles. Arch Gen Psychiatry 44:675–701, 1987

Manu P, Matthews DA, Lane TJ: The mental health of patients with a chief complaint of chronic fatigue: a prospective evaluation and follow up. Arch Intern Med 148:2213–2219, 1988

Manu P, Lane TJ, Matthews DA, et al: Screening for somatization disorder in patients with chronic fatigue. Gen Hosp Psychiatry 11:294–297, 1989

Manu P, Matthews DA, Lane TJ, et al: Screening for treatable mental disorder in patients with chronic fatigue. JAMA (in press)

Othmer E, De Souza C: A screening test for somatization disorder (hysteria). Am J Psychiatry 142:1146–1149, 1985

Robins LN, Helzer JE, Croughan J, et al: The National Institute of Mental Health Diagnostic Interview Schedule: Version III. Department of Health and Human Services, National Institute of Mental Health, Alcohol, Drug Abuse and Mental Health Administration, Rockville, Maryland, May 1981

Rubio-Stipec M, Shrout P, Bird H, et al: Symptom scales of the Diagnostic Interview Schedule: factor results in Hispanic and Anglo samples. J Consult Clin Psychol 1:30–34, 1989

Smith GR, Brown FW: Screening indexes in DSM-III-R somatization disorder. Gen Hosp Psychiatry 12:148–152, 1990

Swartz M, Blazer D, Woodbury M, et al: Somatization disorder in a U.S. southern community: use of a new procedure for analysis of medical classification. Psychol Med 16:595–609, 1986a

Swartz M, Hughes D, George L, et al: Developing a screening test for community studies of somatization disorder. J Psychiatry Res 20:335–343, 1986b

Swartz M, Landerman R, George L, et al: Somatization disorder, in Psychiatric Disorders in America. Edited by Robins LN, Regier DA. New York, Free Press (in press)

Chapter 5

Functional Somatic Syndromes

Laurence J. Kirmayer, M.D., F.R.C.P.(C),
James M. Robbins, Ph.D.

The term *functional* implies a disturbance of physiological function rather than anatomical structure. In clinical usage, *functional* is usually contrasted with *organic* and often carries the added meaning of psychogenic. Stress and psychological conflict are frequently presumed to cause and/or exacerbate functional symptoms. Functional symptoms may then be viewed as somatized expressions of essentially social or psychological problems. However, because the psychosocial determinants of symptoms are difficult to establish with certainty, the assumption that functional symptoms are psychogenic is often unwarranted.

The distinction between functional and organic is rooted in the dualistic ontology of biomedicine: some diseases are more real than others (see Fabrega, Jr., Chapter 9, this volume). Yet, from a psychosomatic perspective, functional disorders are just as real and biological as problems with obvious organic lesions. Functional disorders likely involve physiological disruptions that are too complex or subtle to be reflected in gross structural defects. The hierarchical systems view suggests that the distinction between functional and organic is really one between levels of process and structure: functional disorders may involve abnormal processes occurring in structurally intact organ systems.

In this chapter we summarize studies on the prevalence, symptomatology, and natural history of the most common functional somatic symptoms and syndromes in medical practice. We use this information to address two fundamental problems in current understanding of functional somatic distress:

1. Are psychological factors best understood as causes, consequences, or concomitants of functional somatic distress? The relationship of psychological distress to medically unexplained symptoms remains a complex problem in which studies are often unable to discriminate between psychosocial factors that are causes

of somatic distress, those that simply accompany or co-occur with somatic symptoms (and that may act to exacerbate or maintain distress, help seeking, and disability), and those that are themselves primarily consequences of persistent unexplained somatic symptoms.

2. Are the abridged criteria for functional somatization disorder proposed by Escobar et al. (1989; see also Chapter 4, this volume) likely to classify patients with somatic symptoms confined to one organ system as having "subsyndromal" somatization disorder? Should functional somatization be understood as a single syndrome with mild severity corresponding to the discrete syndromes identified by medical specialists? Alternatively, are functional syndromes distinct and unrelated entities reflecting qualitatively different problems than somatization disorder?

We will present some preliminary results using latent variable modeling to address these questions.

COMMON FUNCTIONAL SOMATIC SYNDROMES

Somatic symptoms of medically unknown origin are common in the community and in most clinical settings (Kellner 1985). Every medical specialty has identified functional syndromes peculiar to its patient population. In doing so, the practitioner, guided by the narrow focus of the specialty, attends to symptoms in one organ system and takes less note of symptoms affecting theoretically unrelated systems. Patients, too, may focus on symptoms they believe are relevant to the concerns of the specialist whom they are consulting, relegating other symptoms to a background of ill-described generalized malaise. Yet the descriptions of the functional somatic syndromes recognized by different medical specialists involve a great deal of symptomatic overlap. Systematic questioning of patients may substantiate even higher degrees of symptom co-occurrence. As will be seen below, three of the most common syndromes share many symptoms and psychopathological profiles and result in similar illness behavior.

Fibromyalgia Syndrome

Fibromyalgia or fibrositis is a syndrome of chronic musculoskeletal aches, pains, and stiffness of unknown etiology (Bennett 1981; Smythe 1980). While recent studies have identified nonspecific immunopathological changes in the muscles of patients with fibromyalgia syndrome (FMS), there are no reliable histological changes and no definite organic pathology has been demonstrated (Goldenberg 1988; McCain and Scudds 1988).

Symptoms involve primarily soft tissues with acute tenderness upon pressure (i.e., tender points) noted at many specific anatomical landmarks, including bony prominences, muscle insertions, and the bodies of many muscles. Other somatic symptoms commonly associated with FMS include nonrestorative sleep (awakening unrefreshed), fatigue, malaise, headache, and, in approximately one-third of patients, symptoms of irritable bowel syndrome (IBS) (Goldenberg 1987; Yunus et al. 1981). Variant criteria for the diagnoses of FMS have been proposed, differing principally in the number of tender points required and the importance of associated symptoms. A recent multicenter study of diagnostic criteria by the American College of Rheumatology evaluated many alternative sets of criteria and derived consensus criteria that discriminated well between FMS patients and other rheumatologic patients at different clinics (Wolfe et al. 1990). The proposed criteria require 1) a history of widespread musculoskeletal pain and 2) pain in 11 of 18 tender point sites on digital palpation. The criteria yielded a sensitivity of 88% and a specificity of 81% measured against rheumatologists' standard diagnostic practice as a gold standard. There was no difference in symptomatology between primary fibromyalgia (without accompanying organic illness) and secondary fibromyalgia (attributed to a preexisting rheumatologic or systemic condition, e.g., rheumatoid arthritis). The committee therefore suggested abolishing the distinction. Further, with these criteria, exclusionary tests for organic disease are not necessary to make a positive diagnosis of FMS.

Syndromes of chronic functional musculoskeletal pain that, with better understanding of pathophysiology, may prove to be related to FMS include myofascial pain, temporomandibular joint dysfunction, chronic idiopathic low back pain, repetitive strain injury, and chronic tension headache (McCain and Scudds 1988).

Prevalence and course. Fibromyalgia is the third most common disorder in rheumatologic practice following osteoarthritis and rheumatoid arthritis. Wolfe and Cathey (1985) found that among 980 consecutive patients attending a private rheumatology clinic, 11% had seven or more tender points and 5% had 12 or more. In a sample of all patients ($N = 1,473$) seen in a private rheumatic disease clinic over a 2½-year period, Wolfe and Cathey (1983) found a prevalence of 3.7% for primary FMS and 12.2% for FMS secondary to other rheumatologic conditions.

FMS symptoms are also common, although underrecognized, in primary care, with an estimated prevalence of 6% (Campbell et al. 1983). There are no reliable estimates of the prevalence of FMS in the community, but FMS is associated with persistent functional disability, and FMS-like symptoms are a common cause of disability and loss of time from work (Cathey et al. 1986).

Pathophysiology. FMS may be associated with a generalized hypersensitivity to sensory stimuli (e.g., see Gerster and Hadj-Djilani 1984), suggesting a central alteration of sensory processing, or with a specific disorder of pain modulation (Goldenberg 1987; Scudds et al. 1987). Some research has suggested an etiologic role for non-REM (Stage 4) sleep deprivation in the production of FMS symptoms. Patients with FMS have disturbed sleep architecture with a lessening of Stage 4 delta-wave sleep (Moldofsky et al. 1975) and, in some cases, sleep-related myoclonus (Moldofsky et al. 1984). When healthy volunteers were selectively deprived of Stage 4 sleep in the laboratory, they developed muscular aches and tender points typical of FMS (Moldofsky et al. 1976). These intriguing results have not been replicated but suggest a possible common pathway in the genesis of FMS symptoms in which major depression, anxiety, or physical deconditioning might give rise to FMS through a disruption of normal sleep.

Moldofsky et al. (1976) found that athletic subjects in good cardiovascular condition tended not to experience FMS symptoms in response to sleep deprivation. Other studies have confirmed that FMS patients tend to have poor fitness and that cardiovascular conditioning affords protection or relief from symptoms of FMS (Bennett et al. 1989). Antidepressants have been reported to be useful in FMS and other chronic pain syndromes in doses usually insufficient to treat depression, perhaps because of independent effects on pain modulation or sleep physiology (Carette et al. 1986).

Psychopathology. A psychogenic cause has been repeatedly proposed for FMS, although results from studies to date have been inconsistent. Payne et al. (1982) studied 30 hospitalized FMS patients and compared them with patients having rheumatoid arthritis and other chronic arthritic diseases. They found that the FMS patients were a very heterogeneous group, with elevated scores on six Minnesota Multiphasic Personality Inventory (MMPI) scales, but reaching pathological levels on only two scales: hypochondriasis and hysteria. Other researchers have found similar results with ambulatory FMS patients, suggesting that about one-third of FMS patients display abnormal scores on MMPI hypochondriasis or hysteria scales, about one-third are somatically preoccupied, and about one-third give no evidence of psychological disturbance (Ahles et al. 1984; Wolfe et al. 1984). Similar patterns of elevated MMPI scores are also found among patients with rheumatoid arthritis and other organic illnesses, and may reflect levels of somatic distress rather than psychopathology (Pincus et al. 1986).

It has been suggested that FMS is a form of somatized depression in which the preoccupation with physical symptoms diverts the attention of both patient and physician away from the affective and psychosocial aspect of suffering (Blumer and Heilbronn 1982). Hudson et al. (1985) administered the DSM-III Diagnostic Interview Schedule (DIS) to 31 patients meeting the criteria of Yunus et al. (1981) for FMS. Seventy-one percent of patients had a history of affective disorder, while 26% were currently suffering from an episode of major affective disorder. A separate family history interview revealed a significantly greater incidence of major affective disorder among the relatives of FMS patients than among comparison groups of families of patients with rheumatoid arthritis and schizophrenia. A later extension by Goldenberg (1986) of the original Hudson et al. sample found less evidence of current depression, although depression was still significantly more common in the past histories of FMS patients compared with rheumatoid arthritic control subjects.

Our own study failed to confirm a high prevalence of current or lifetime major depression in FMS patients. Only 20% of FMS patients had lifetime history of major depression—a level not significantly different from a comparison group of patients with rheumatoid arthritis (Kirmayer et al. 1988). Dysthymia was actually more common among rheumatoid arthritic patients. Also, there was no difference between groups on the Center for Epidemiologic Studies Depression (CES-D) scale (Roberts and Vernon 1983), a measure of depressive symptomatology—a negative finding also reported by Ahles et al. (1987) utilizing the Zung Depression Scale. At 1-year follow-up, FMS patients were more likely to report having a lot of trouble with nerves or nervousness in the preceding 12 months.

Illness behavior. Pain, depression, and disability make separate contributions to FMS patients' estimates of the severity of their illness (Hawley et al. 1988). In a sample of 22 patients meeting stringent criteria for FMS, identified by screening in a primary setting, Clark et al. (1985) found no significant differences among control subjects drawn from the same general medical outpatient population on the Beck Depression Inventory, the Spielberger State and Trait Anxiety Inventory, and the Symptom Checklist-90-Revised (SCL-90-R). These patients had not sought help specifically for their FMS, suggesting that the observed associations between psychological distress and FMS may be related to help-seeking behavior.

In our study of patients attending a rheumatologic practice, FMS patients were significantly more likely than rheumatoid arthritic patients to report medically unexplained somatic symptoms of all types, including cardiovascular, psychosexual, and pseudoneurological symptoms (Kirmayer et al. 1988). FMS patients had seen three times as many physicians for their symptoms prior to consulting the rheumatologist. When joint surgery was excluded, FMS patients had undergone significantly more surgical procedures than had patients with rheumatoid arthritis. FMS patients reported comparable levels of pain and social disability but markedly less physical disability than rheumatoid arthritic patients. There were no differences between FMS and rheumatoid arthritic patients on measures of introspectiveness, body focus, somatic illness worry, somatic versus psychological symptom attribution, or help-seeking propensity (J. M. Robbins, L. J. Kirmayer, M. A. Kapusta, 1987, unpublished data). Interestingly, disability correlated with illness worry for FMS patients but not for rheumatoid arthritic patients (Robbins et al. 1990b). Some FMS patients may restrict their physical and social activity because of high levels of illness worry that are maintained by the lack of a generally accepted medical explanation for their condition.

An epidemic of chronic upper limb pain, termed repetitive strain injury (RSI) syndrome has recently been reported among Australian workers (Hall and Morrow 1988; Miller and Topliss 1988). While physical strain related to specific occupational tasks is a plausible cause of muscular pain, the chronicity and disability of RSI syndrome appear to be related to the effects of the diagnostic label on individuals' perception of common symptoms in concert with the validating response of the medical and compensation systems.

Irritable Bowel Syndrome

Irritable bowel is a syndrome of abdominal pain, distension, and alteration of bowel habits (Drossman et al. 1977). Until recently, clinicians have viewed IBS as a diagnosis of exclusion, ruling out organic bowel disease with extensive investigations that included blood tests, sigmoidoscopy, air-contrast barium enema, and upper gastrointestinal tract radiography and/or endoscopy, stool cultures, parasite studies, and lactose tolerance tests. Kruis et al. (1984) found that a combination of symptom questions, physical examination, and minimal basic blood tests (erythrocyte sedimentation rate, white cell count, and hemoglobin) could distinguish IBS from organic disease with a sensitivity of 83% and a specificity of 97% compared with the usual extensive workup. Manning et al. (1978) provided evidence that IBS could be distinguished from organic gastrointestinal disorders solely on the basis of detailed information on symptomatology. These authors noted that clinicians did not routinely collect this symptom information. In a study of gastrointestinal patients and healthy control subjects, Talley et al. (1990) found that the criteria of Manning et al. were moderately specific but not sensitive to IBS. The inclusion of one additional criterion, "stools that were loose and watery," improved the accuracy of the Manning criteria. A factor analytic study has also confirmed the existence of a pattern of symptoms consistent with IBS and not correlated with lactose intolerance (Whitehead et al. 1990). Taken together, these studies suggest that it is possible to achieve a diagnostic accuracy for IBS of greater than 80% purely with questions about symptoms. Recently, an international commission of established researchers and experts proposed consensus criteria for the diagnosis of IBS (Thompson et al. 1989): 1) abdominal pain that is relieved with defecation or associated with a change in frequency or consistency of stools; and/or 2) disturbed defecation (defined as altered stool frequency, altered stool form, straining or urgency, feeling of incomplete evacuation, or passage of mucus), usually associated with 3) bloating or a feeling of abdominal distension.

Prevalence and course. Surveys using self-reported diagnoses of "spastic colon" or irritable bowel yield a community prevalence for IBS of 2.9% (Sandler 1990). IBS symptoms are reported by 8% to 22% of the general population, although only a small proportion of people seek medical help (Sandler et al. 1984; Whitehead et al. 1982). In Britain and Canada, up to 20% of suffers may seek help, owing, perhaps, to the greater accessibility of medical care (Thompson and Heaton 1980). IBS is the second leading cause of work absenteeism in North America, and IBS-related complaints constitute about 10% of all general practitioner visits and account for 40% to 50% of all referrals to gastroenterologists (Sammons and Karoly 1987).

Pathophysiology. Food intolerance and dietary fiber deficiency do not seem to account for the majority of clinical cases of IBS (Read 1987). IBS symptoms do not closely follow objective indicators of bowel function (Oettlé and Heaton 1986). Disturbed gut motility has been proposed as a cause of IBS and other functional syndromes, including esophageal spasm and dyspepsia (Clouse 1988). Pain and emotional distress can provoke changes in gut motility in both healthy individuals and IBS patients (Welgan et al. 1985). The abnormalities of gastrointestinal motility seen in IBS are similar to patterns seen in healthy subjects under stress and in patients with psychoneurotic disorders without gastrointestinal symptoms (Latimer 1983). Recent studies of IBS patients reporting increased tonic levels of colon activity (Welgan et al. 1985) or suppression and irregular contractile activity with mental stress (Kumar and Wingate 1985) require replication.

Psychopathology. Major psychosocial problems and stressful life events have been reported in 70% to 80% of IBS patients (Sammons and Karoly 1987). Hislop (1971) found significantly higher frequencies of marital disharmony and financial and occupational stress in IBS patients compared with matched control subjects. In a study of 135 consecutive referrals to gastroenterology clinics, severely threatening life events were experienced by 57% of 79 patients with a functional gastrointestinal disorder compared with 23% of patients with organic gastrointestinal disease and 15% of a community sample (Craig and Brown 1984). In a study using similar measures of stressful life events and the Present State Examination for psychiatric morbidity, Ford et al. (1987) found that psychiatric disorders and/or anxiety-provoking situations preceded symptom onset in 32 of 48 patients with functional gastrointestinal disorders but not in any of 16 patients with organic disease. Life situations alone did not appear to induce functional disorders unless they first gave rise to an anxiety state.

Several studies with various methodologies have reported higher frequencies of symptoms of anxiety, depression, and unspecified psychiatric morbidity in IBS subjects compared with healthy control subjects (Sammons and Karoly 1987; Walker et al. 1990). Hislop (1971) found symptoms of depression, fatigue, and insomnia in 50% to 60% of a sample of IBS patients. Studies using Research Diagnostic Criteria (RDC) have reported psychiatric disorders in 78% to 92% of IBS patients—predominantly depression, hysteria, and "unspecified disorders" (Liss et al. 1973; Young et al. 1976). Whitehead et al. (1980) found elevated levels of anxiety, depression, and hostility in IBS patients, but these appeared to be unrelated to changes in colonic motility or severity of symptoms. Toner et al. (1990) found that 43% of a sample of 21 patients with IBS met DSM-III criteria for major depression in the last year. Compared with a matched group of psychiatric outpatients with depression, the IBS patients with depression did not view themselves as depressed on a measure of self-schema. Unfortunately, psychiatric patients with a history of IBS were excluded from the study, so that it is not possible to determine whether the differences in self-schema stem from differences in help-seeking and in how patients describe themselves in a specific clinic context or are more directly related to the different phenomenology of depression with and without concurrent IBS.

Illness behavior. Most people with IBS symptoms in the community do not seek medical help. In a well-designed study comparing IBS patients with persons with IBS who had not sought medical help and with healthy control subjects, Drossman et al. (1988) found that only the IBS patients had evidence of increased psychopathology with elevated MMPI hypochondriasis, depression, hysteria, psychasthenia, and schizophrenia scores as well as increased hypochondriacal worry on the Illness Behavior Questionnaire. IBS nonpatients had scores that, while intermediate between those of patients and healthy control subjects, were not significantly different from those of healthy control subjects. There was some indirect evidence that IBS nonpatients were better able than IBS patients to cope with stressful life events and somatic symptoms. Two other studies have confirmed that elevated levels of psychopathology are found among IBS patients but not among IBS sufferers in the community (Smith et al. 1990; Whitehead et al. 1988). Thus, psychopathology appears to be associated not with IBS per se but with an increased propensity to seek medical care.

IBS patients who seek help often report many other nonspecific somatic complaints, including headache, fatigue, dysmenorrhea, and dysuria (Drossman et al. 1977). Using RDC criteria, Young et al. (1976) diagnosed hysteria in 17% of 29 consecutive IBS patients compared with only 3% of 33 control subjects. Welch et al. (1985) found higher levels of somatic symptomatology with the SCL-90 in both IBS outpatients and community "nonreporters" with symptoms of IBS compared with healthy control subjects.

In a telephone survey of 832 people, Whitehead et al. (1982) found that people with symptoms of IBS were more likely than those without symptoms to be hospitalized for acute illnesses, to make more doctor visits, and to perceive illnesses as being more serious. Twenty-one percent of IBS subjects reported missing work or a social obligation more than 4 days a year compared with 9% of the non-IBS group.

Retrospective studies of IBS patients suggest differences in childhood illness experience that may help account for increased help seeking. Whitehead et al. (1982) reported that people with IBS symptoms were more likely than people with peptic ulcer disease or no gastrointestinal symptoms to have received parental favors or gifts as children when ill. Lowman et al. (1987), comparing patients and nonpatients having IBS with asymptomatic control subjects, found evidence for increased childhood gastrointestinal illness experience, parental attention for illness, frequent school absences, and doctor visits only among the patient group. Children with IBS have been found to have higher levels of anxiety and functional somatic symptoms, and a family history of abdominal pain or other gastrointestinal problems (Apley 1975). An epidemiologic study of 308 preschool children found that mothers of children with recurrent stomachaches were more likely to be depressed, to report marital difficulties, and to report their own health as poor (Zuckerman et al. 1987).

Chronic Fatigue Syndrome

There has been much recent interest in the possibility that certain acute viral infections may result in a prolonged postviral syndrome characterized by easy fatigability, muscular weakness, myalgias, and mild cognitive impairment. Because many authorities continue to doubt the existence of the syndrome, there are no generally agreed-upon criteria for diagnosis. In an effort to promote further research, a restrictive case definition of chronic fatigue syndrome (CFS) has been proposed (Holmes et al. 1988). This definition requires two major criteria: 1) new onset of debilitating fatigue, persisting or relapsing for at least 6 months; and 2) no evidence of any other clinical condition that can produce such symptoms. In addition, the criteria require at least 6 of 11 minor symptoms or signs, including mild fever, sore throat, painful cervical or axillary lymph nodes, generalized muscle weakness, myalgia, prolonged fatigue after exercise, headache, arthralgias, neuropsychological symptoms (e.g., photophobia, irritability, difficulty thinking, depression), and sleep disturbance. Physical signs—which must be documented by a physician on at least two separate occasions at least 1 month apart—include low-grade fever, nonexudative pharyngitis, and palpable or tender cervical or axillary lymph nodes. The neuropsychiatric symptoms of CFS may not be associated with objective abnormalities on neuropsychological testing (Altay et al. 1990). The inclusion of physical signs is intended to aid in the distinction between CFS and other nonspecific causes of fatigue. To date, however, most studies have employed more liberal criteria, relying primarily on the presence of medically unexplained chronic fatigue to make the diagnosis. Syndromes of generalized malaise closely related to CFS include neurasthenia, neurocirculatory asthenia, chronic brucellosis, hypoglycemia, benign or myalgic encephalomyelitis, "20th-century disease," total allergy syndrome or multiple chemical sensitivity, and chronic candidiasis (Greenberg 1990; Kleinman 1986; Simon et al. 1990; Stewart 1990; Stewart and Raskin 1985; Wessely 1990a, 1990b).

Prevalence and course. Community surveys in Britain and North America find that more than 20% of adults report feeling "tired all the time" (cf. Chen 1986; Wessely 1990b). Fatigue is the seventh most common presenting complaint in primary care medicine in the United States (National Center for Health Statistics 1978). A survey of 500 unselected patients attending a teaching-hospital primary care clinic found that 21% were suffering from symptoms consistent with CFS

(Buchwald et al. 1987b). The mean duration of fatigue was 16 months (range 6 to 458 months), and 28% of the patients had been completely bedridden at some time because of the severity of their fatigue. Sixty percent of the fatigue patients reported that their symptoms had caused considerable stress at work or at home. Common associated symptoms included depression or mood changes, difficulty sleeping, difficulty concentrating, anxiety, nausea, stomachache, diarrhea, odd sensations in skin, and joint pain.

Manu et al. (1988) applied the proposed CFS diagnostic criteria to 135 patients with chief complaints of persistent fatigue attending an internal medicine fatigue clinic. Only six patients met the restrictive criteria. One-fourth of the patients had insufficient symptoms or signs to meet the criteria, while 67% of the patients had current psychiatric disorders (an exclusion criterion in the restrictive case definition). This study makes it clear that, with the restrictive case definition, CFS is a rare condition in primary care and cannot account for the frequency of fatigue as a presenting complaint.

Symptoms of CFS are common in other functional somatic syndromes. Buchwald et al. (1987a) studied 50 patients with primary FMS and found a high prevalence of recurrent sore throat, rashes, adenopathy, and low-grade fevers as well as chronic cough. However, viral antibody titers were not significantly elevated compared with those of matched control subjects.

CFS is usually described as a chronic disorder with a poor prognosis. Although patients do not seem to suffer from excess medical morbidity, they do tend to report persistent work and social disability (Kroenk et al. 1988; Wessely 1990b).

Pathophysiology. The pathophysiology of fatigue is poorly understood. With physical exertion, changes occur in muscle and at the neuromuscular junction, but reported fatigue correlates poorly with these peripheral changes, suggesting that the central nervous system and psychological processes play a key role (Kennedy 1988). Similarly, anxious patients who hyperventilate may experience fatigue, but this characteristic does not correlate with changes in muscle electromyographic activity or CO_2 levels (Folgering and Snik 1988).

Fatigue, myalgias, and malaise accompany many viral illnesses, and it has been proposed that CFS might reflect a chronic infection. Attention has focussed on Epstein-Barr virus, which can give rise to a chronic infection that is, however, usually much more severe than CFS (Straus 1988). The possible existence of a milder form of chronic mononucleosis cannot be ruled out, although virological studies have been equivocal, with comparable levels of viral antibodies being found in both affected individuals and healthy control subjects, and with many CFS patients having no serological evidence of infection (Buchwald et al. 1987b; Holmes et al. 1987; Tobi and Straus 1985). Exogenously administered interferon produces symptoms of fatigue, including slowness, drowsiness, and confusion (McDonald et al. 1987). Viral infection may contribute to CFS as a nonspecific precipitant of immune dysfunction (Lloyd et al. 1988). In studies to date, however, the severity of symptoms in CFS does not correlate with measures of immunological function (Straus 1988).

Psychopathology. Clinicians have attributed chronic fatigue to a wide range of psychiatric disorders, including depression, anxiety, adjustment disorder, alcoholism, or even to a "stressful life-style." Taerk et al. (1987) found that 16 of 24 patients with CFS had current major depression, while 50% had a history of affective disorder prior to the onset of CFS. Employing the DIS, Kruesi et al. (1989) at the National Institute of Mental Health (NIMH) found that 75% of a sample of 28 patients meeting the Centers for Disease Control criteria for CFS had lifetime histories of major psychiatric disorders—primarily depression (46%), dysthymia, and simple phobia. In only two cases did the CFS precede the onset of depression, while for 10 patients, psychiatric disorders occurred prior to or concurrently with the onset of CFS symptoms. Two female subjects met DSM-III criteria for somatization disorder. When physical symptoms related to CFS were scored as indicative of psychiatric distress, two more subjects reached criteria for somatization disorder, for a total of four subjects (14.6%).

Using a similar methodology, Manu et al. (1989) studied 100 patients attending a fatigue clinic in a general medical outpatient setting. Seventy-seven patients had one or more lifetime psychiatric diagnoses, and 59 had current disorders, including major depression ($n = 36$), somatization disorder ($n = 10$), and dysthymia ($n = 6$). An additional five patients met criteria for somatization disorder at 6-month follow-up. Organic causes found for fatigue in five patients included seizure disorder, obstructive sleep apnea, bronchial asthma, and polymyalgia rheumatica. Several somatic symptoms—including pain in extremities, joint pain, chest pain, other pain, shortness of breath, blurred vision, muscle weakness or paralysis, and sexual indifference—were reported significantly more frequently by the CFS patients with somatization disorder than by those with other psychiatric diagnoses.

In a careful study at a neurological hospital, Wessely and Powell (1989) compared 47 patients with unexplained chronic fatigue with two control groups: one of patients with peripheral neuromuscular diseases causing fatigue (myasthenia gravis, myopathy, Guillain-Barré syndrome, and genetic or metabolic muscle disorders) and a second control group of psychiatric inpatients with current major depression. Both the CFS and depressed groups reported significantly more physical and, especially, mental fatigue than the neuromuscular group. Only the CFS and depressed patients reported that mental effort could precipitate their fatigue. Seventy-two percent of the CFS patients met RDC criteria for a current psychiatric disorder (modified to exclude fatigue as a criterion)—primarily major depression (47%) and somatization disorder (15%). Forty-three percent of the CFS patients had a past psychiatric history. The highest levels of somatic symptoms were reported by the CFS group, but only headache, eyestrain, tremor, and muscle pain at rest were significantly more frequent in the CFS patients than in the depressed patients. In fact, most of the symptoms held to be specific for postviral fatigue—including hypersomnia, sensitivity to noise, gastrointestinal disturbance, and muscle pain after exercise—were equally common among depressed and CFS patients.

Illness behavior. Wessely and Powell (1989) found that the major difference between their CFS patients and depressed controls was in symptom attribution. The majority of CFS patients, including those with diagnosable major depressions, believed they had a physical illness, which was in contrast to the depressed inpatients, who viewed their illness as psychological. The CFS patients displayed lower levels of guilt and self-blame than did depressed control subjects. Physical attributions of emotional distress may protect CFS patients from some of the distressing psychological symptoms of depression at the same time as they may lead to ineffective help seeking. Epidemic forms of CFS-like conditions have been described (e.g., Royal Free disease, Iceland disease, epidemic neuromyasthenia) that may reflect "mass hysteria"—that is, social processes, including heightened medical attention, that result in the amplification and pathological attribution of nonspecific somatic symptoms arising from disparate causes including social stress and psychiatric morbidity (Wessely 1990a, 1990b; cf. Pennebaker and Watson, Chapter 2, this volume).

LATENT-VARIABLE MODELS OF SOMATIC DISTRESS

A striking feature of the functional syndromes described above is their high degree of overlap in symptomatology. Although in each case a core group of symptoms has been selected as the defining characteristic, patients with FMS, IBS, and CFS share many associated symptoms. While it is certainly possible that the functional somatic syndromes represent distinct disorders with their own pathophysiology and natural history, the overlap in symptomatology raises the possibility that a single somatization disorder underlies all these syndromes. Medical specialists who focus on a limited range of somatic distress may identify these disorders as discrete by discounting co-occurring symptoms in other bodily systems.

Swartz et al. (1986) have used the latent structure technique of grade-of-membership analysis to study whether somatization symptoms naturally cluster into syndromes when no prior assumptions have been made about the interrelationships among symptoms. Using data from the Piedmont Epidemiologic Catchment Area (ECA) study, seven symptom clusters were derived. Of those, one cluster included many symptoms of somatization disorder, offering validation for the existence of DSM-III somatization disorder as a naturally occurring diagnostic entity. Other clusters grouped together gastrointestinal symptoms (including core symptoms of IBS), cardiovascular symptoms (including many associated with panic disorder), and affective and somatic symptoms of depression. A further cluster comprised symptoms of musculoskeletal pain, weakness, and conversion symptoms. These results suggest that functional somatic syndromes similar to IBS, FMS, and somatic anxiety and depression exist as discrete entities along with a more general construct of somatization disorder.

In an attempt to further explore alternative latent-variable models of functional somatic syndromes, we used the statistical technique of confirmatory factor analysis (Robbins et al. 1990a).[1] As with all latent structure procedures, this technique assumes that some underlying constructs—referred to as *latent variables*—cannot be directly measured. Knowledge about these latent variables can be gained indirectly through their effects on observed variables (Long 1983). In confirmatory factor analysis, we hypothesize latent variables and their relationship to observed variables, compute a set of correlations based on the hypothesized relationships, then test these correlations against the observed correlations to determine whether the model is a good fit to the actual data. If the fit is poor, the model can be respecified and tested again. This recursive process can uncover more adequate models to account for the relationship between observed variables. The statistical method we used (i.e., LISREL) produces biased estimates of parameters with dichotomous and skewed data like that available from the DIS (Ethington 1987). Accordingly, the results presented below must be viewed as rough estimates that require replication with statistical methods that employ distribution-

[1]The research reported in this section was aided by a grant from the Conseil québecois de la recherche sociale. We thank Sherri Tepper and Blair Wheaton for their contributions to the statistical analysis.

free estimation procedures and that allow for dichotomous observed variables (e.g., LISCOMP [Muthen 1984]).

Our sample consisted of 698 patients attending two general hospital family-medicine clinics in Montreal on a self-initiated visit. The mean age was 44.4 years (SD = 16.6); the mean number of years of education was 12.5 (SD = 4.0), and the average household income was $24,423. The sex ratio of patients in the sample (42% male) was comparable to the ratio of all patients eligible for inclusion (45% male). Further characteristics of the sample are described in Chapter 6 (this volume).

All patients were interviewed by trained lay interviewers using the DIS, version 3 (Robins et al. 1981). The somatization section of the DIS determines whether each symptom was sufficiently severe to cause a visit to the doctor or to interfere with life or activities, and whether the symptom occurred only while taking alcohol, drugs, or medication, or only as a result of a physical illness or injury. Symptoms are scored as functional only if they were not the result of injury or drug use, and if no plausible organic diagnosis was given by a doctor. To distinguish between a valid medical explanation for somatic symptoms and an invalid one, we conducted a medical audit of the DIS protocols. Although in the absence of physical examination and laboratory investigations it is not possible to fully distinguish functional symptoms from organic disease, the DIS identifies symptoms that are more likely to be functional than those identified simply by self-report checklists typically used in epidemiologic surveys. While it is the best available instrument for the study of functional somatic symptoms, the DIS has a number of serious limitations: it does not canvass the full range of symptoms associated with the common functional somatic syndromes; it does not distinguish between acute episodes and chronic illness; and it does not inquire into the temporal co-occurrence of somatic symptoms. These limitations would tend to exaggerate the degree of association between symptoms that, in fact, were acute and occurred at different times. The models we present thus approximate an upper bound on the degree of association between symptoms and syndromes.

We began the analysis by identifying 23 somatic symptoms from the somatization and depression sections of the DIS that corresponded to the published definitions of three common functional somatic syndromes—FMS, IBS, and CFS—as well as to the hypothetical syndromes of somatic depression and anxiety. We then proceeded to estimate progressively more elaborate latent-variable models.

The first model examined whether the symptoms associated with FMS, CFS, and IBS, as well as the physical symptoms known to be associated with depressive or anxiety disorders, might be due to a single underlying construct, akin to negative affectivity (cf. Pennebaker and Watson, Chapter 2, this volume) or the somatization trait posited by Escobar (1987). With this single construct model, there was a statistically significant difference between the theoretically predicted and the observed correlations, suggesting that, while all of the functional symptoms tend to co-occur, a single construct is insufficient to account for the covariation among symptoms.

In the second model we hypothesized two latent variables underlying somatic distress: one encompassing the vegetative symptoms of depression plus chronic pain symptoms (Blumer and Heilbronn 1982) and a second reflecting the autonomic and somatomotor manifestations of generalized anxiety and/or pain disorder. A symptom was assigned to somatic depression or somatic anxiety if it was a core symptom of the DSM-III-R description of the disorder or if it was usually described as a symptom of only one syndrome. The results largely confirmed the conventional association between mood disorder and somatic symptoms, with a few interesting exceptions. Abdominal pain, initially hypothesized to be closer to a depressive "pain-prone disorder," was found to occur more consistently with other somatic symptoms of anxiety than with depression. Weakness, initially considered a symptom consistent with only somatic depression, was found to occur as well with somatic anxiety. Although this two-construct model fit the data better than did the single-construct model, the covariation among observed variables was still poorly reproduced. Of course, anxiety and depression are related and often difficult to distinguish even when affective symptoms are prominent (Eaton and Ritter 1988). This may make the recognition of somatic syndromes of depression and anxiety, in which affective and cognitive symptoms may be "masked" or muted, yet more difficult to detect.

The third model tested the hypothesis that the covariation of somatic symptoms could be accounted for by five latent constructs: CFS, FMS, IBS, somatic depression, and somatic anxiety. Symptoms were assigned as observed indicators of each condition according to their current clinical descriptions as summarized above. The resulting five-factor model appears in Figure 5-1. The latent-variable constructs are labeled FM, CF, and IB to distinguish them from the actual clinical syndromes FMS, CFS, and IBS, which they can only approximate because of the intrinsic limitations of a purely interview-based diagnostic method like the DIS.

Several of the conventional associations between symptoms and syndromes were contradicted by the data from the third model. Constipation was found not to covary with other symptoms of the somatic depression construct. Similarly, joint pain and extremity pain, described in the literature as minor symptoms of CFS, were not associated with the CF construct. Nausea, which was initially not identified as a core symptom of IBS, was found to be a good indicator of the IB construct.

The five-construct model provided a much better statistical fit to the data. Although the χ^2 value (402) remained significant (df = 215, $p < .001$), the ratio of χ^2 to degrees of freedom was 1.86, indicating reasonable fit (Carmines and McIver 1981).

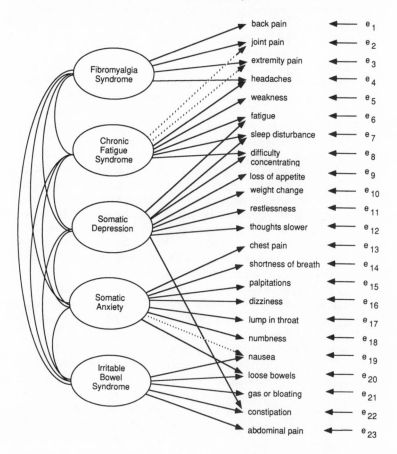

Figure 5-1. Confirmatory factor analytical model of functional somatic syndromes among family medicine patients. Dashed lines denote effects hypothesized but not confirmed.

The five-factor model provides evidence for the convergent validity of the clinically described functional somatic syndromes. Symptoms commonly reported as occurring with FMS, CFS, and IBS, or as somatic manifestations of depression and anxiety, were found to covary more within syndromes than between syndromes. This does not mean, however, that these syndromes occur in isolation. Correlations among the five latent variables were all above .4 and in one case (CF and somatic anxiety) reached .8. Only for FM and somatic depression was the correlation weak.

To further explore the nature of these latent variables, we compared patients who scored in the top 10% cutoff for each latent functional syndrome with patients who did not score above the cutoff on any syndrome. Consistent with other reports (Buchwald et al. 1987b; Drossman et al. 1977; Goldenberg 1987), women were overrepresented among patients with functional syndromes, although not significantly overrepresented among those patients above the 10% cutoff on FM and CF. Patients high on any of the latent syndrome measures were significantly more likely to have presented to the family-medicine clinic with psychosocial complaints. These complaints included feelings of being stressed or nervous, sadness, trouble concentrating, family problems, or troubles at work. Lifetime DIS diagnoses of major depression and anxiety disorders were significantly more frequent among all syndrome groups except FM. Current DIS diagnoses of depression or anxiety were significantly higher for all groups. Half of the CF group had a history of major depression. Patients above the cutoff on the fibromyalgia measure were less likely to have received DIS diagnoses of major depression or anxiety than were patients in other syndrome groups.

Pure types of syndromes were less likely to occur than mixed types. CF and somatic depression, in particular, rarely occur without the presence of at least one other cluster of functional symptoms. By contrast, of patients above the 10% cutoff for FMS-like symptoms, almost half had only that syndrome.

In a final model we analyzed the associations between disturbed affect and the syndrome latent variables identified in the five-factor solution to attempt to determine whether the syndromes themselves were specifically associated with depressed or anxious mood (whether or not the mood disturbance was part of a full-fledged mood or anxiety disorder). DIS items recording a history of sadness for 2 weeks or more, and whether subjects considered themselves to be a nervous person, were used to predict each of the five syndrome latent variables. Sadness was only a modest predictor of CF, somatic anxiety, and IB and was not related to FM. Nervousness was most strongly associated with somatic depression and somatic anxiety, and also predicted CF, IB, and FM.

CONCLUSIONS

Psychosocial factors may contribute to the pathogenesis of functional somatic symptoms. An increased frequency of recent negative life events has been found in patients presenting with a variety of acute functional somatic symptoms, including abdominal pain, noncardiac chest pain, and pseudoneurological or conversion symptoms (Creed et al. 1988; Mayou 1989; Raskin et al. 1966; Robinson et al. 1988; Roll and Theorell 1987; Scaloubaca et al. 1988). Because most of these studies compared only clinical samples, it is not possible to ascertain whether the stressful events cause the somatic symptoms, precipitate help seeking, or are simply reported more frequently by patients searching for an explanation for medically unexplained illness. For chronic functional somatic syndromes the etiologic role of life events is much less clear, although enduring social stresses may contribute to a poor outcome (Drossman et al. 1988; Jensen 1988).

Clinical studies suggest a high prevalence of psychiatric disorders in patients with functional somatic syndromes. The association is strongest for CFS: even when strict criteria requiring physical signs of viral infection are employed, most patients with CFS meet criteria for a depressive or anxiety disorder. The association with major psychiatric disorders is less dramatic for IBS and FMS, although there is ample evidence that both syndromes are exacerbated by dysphoric mood.

Community surveys of functional somatic syndromes are difficult to conduct, since in the absence of extensive history, physical examination, and laboratory investigations, it is often not possible to rule out alternate diagnoses, including organic disease. Where community surveys have been attempted, much weaker correlations have been found between psychiatric morbidity and functional somatic syndromes. The association between psychiatric disorders and functional somatic syndromes seen in clinical samples may be inflated compared with those found in the community, because coexisting psychiatric disorders compel many people with functional somatic syndromes, who might otherwise cope with their symptoms, to seek medical help.

For patients the distinctive feature of functional somatic syndromes is that their illness lacks objectively verifiable indicators of pathology. Consequently, patients with these syndromes may suffer added worry, self-doubt, and public censure due to the ambiguity or "unreality" of their illness. This negation of their experience may give rise to particular forms of illness behavior—such as the adamant rejection of psychological causation—in an effort to obtain medical and social validation for their suffering. These patterns of illness behavior are probably social consequences rather than causes of functional somatic syndromes.

We applied latent-variable analysis to explore the relationship between the functional somatic symptoms recorded with the DIS in a sample of family-medicine patients. While the results of our latent-variable modeling must be considered tentative because of the methodological limitations in the data and analytic procedures, we found that the pattern of symptom reporting among patients was better characterized by several distinct functional syndromes than by a single somatization disorder. With modifications to the DIS to collect more complete data on relevant symptoms, their duration, and their co-occurrence, latent-structure methods can be used to suggest refinements in diagnostic categories and etiologic investigation.

Our results are relevant to the recent attempts of Escobar and coworkers (see Chapter 4, this volume) to develop abridged diagnostic criteria for somatization disorder. The threshold for distinguishing between patients with isolated functional somatic syndromes and patients with somatization disorder is, at present, entirely arbitrary. Our findings suggest that, with the proposed criteria of four unexplained symptoms for men and six for women (Somatic Symptom Index [SSI 4,6]), many people with a single discrete functional somatic syndrome would be classified as "somatizers." Lumping together individuals with unexplained distress limited to a single functional system and those who experience multiple forms of somatic distress over multiple bodily systems may obscure etiologic factors unique to distinct forms of functional somatic distress.

The evidence reviewed in this chapter suggests that psychiatric disorder may be a cause, concomitant, and consequence of functional somatic distress. While a large proportion of patients with functional somatic syndromes attending medical clinics display clinically significant psychiatric comorbidity, community surveys tend to find that these syndromes are very prevalent and not always associated with increased levels of psychological disturbance. Many functional somatic syndrome symptoms may arise from the direct transduction of psychosocial and physical stress into physiological dysfunction. In these cases, major psychiatric disorders, as well as milder cognitive or affective disturbances, may not play a role in symptom production. People with subclinical or mild functional somatic syndromes may not come to medical attention unless they also experience other incitements to seek help, such as life stress, concomitant depression, or illness worry. The clinician is then faced with at least two distinct problems: physiological dysfunction giving rise to somatic symptoms, and psychiatric distress that exacerbates symptoms, undermines patients' ability to cope with somatic discomfort, and compels help-seeking behavior. Effective diagnosis and treatment must address both of these dimensions of illness experience. The techniques of behavioral medicine allow the clinician to directly address somatic distress through relaxation training, contingency management, cognitive interventions, or hypnosis. Patients who feel their somatic symptoms are being taken seriously and partially alleviated through these techniques are generally more willing to accept treatment of any associated psychiatric disorder and to alter maladaptive illness behavior.

REFERENCES

Ahles TA, Yunus MB, Riley SD, et al: Psychological factors associated with primary fibromyalgia. Arthritis Rheum 27:1101–1106, 1984

Ahles TA, Yunus MB, Masi AT: Is chronic pain a variant of depressive disease? The case of primary fibromyalgia syndrome. Pain 29:105–111, 1987

Altay HT, Toner BB, Brooker H, et al: The neuropsychological dimensions of postinfectious neuromyasthenia (chronic fatigue syndrome): a preliminary report. Int J Psychiatry Med 20:141–149, 1990

Apley J: The Child With Abdominal Pains, 2nd Edition. Oxford, UK, Blackwell, 1975

Bennett RM: Fibrositis: misnomer for a common rheumatic disorder. West J Med 134:405–413, 1981

Bennett RM, Clark, SR, Goldberg L, et al: Aerobic fitness in patients with fibrositis: a controlled study of respiratory gas exchange and ^{133}Xenon clearance from exercising muscle. Arthritis Rheum 32:454–460, 1989

Blumer D, Heilbronn M: Chronic pain as a variant of depressive disease. J Nerv Ment Dis 170:381–406, 1982

Buchwald D, Goldenberg DL, Sullivan JL, et al: The "chronic, active Epstein-Barr virus infection" syndrome and primary fibromyalgia. Arthritis Rheum 30:1132–1136, 1987a

Buchwald D, Sullivan JL, Komaroff AL: Frequency of "chronic, active Epstein-Barr virus infection" in a general medical practice. JAMA 257:2303–2307, 1987b

Campbell SM, Clark S, Tindall EA, et al: Clinical characteristics of fibrositis,

I: a "blinded," controlled study of symptoms and tender points. Arthritis Rheum 26:817–824, 1983

Carette S, McCain GA, Bell DA, et al. Evaluation of amitriptyline in primary fibrositis. Arthritis Rheum 29:655–659, 1986

Carmines EG, McIver JP: Analyzing models with unobserved variables: analysis of covariance structures, in Social Measurement: Current Issues. Edited by Bohrnstedt GW, Borgatta EF. Beverly Hills, CA, Sage, 1981, pp 65–115

Cathey MA, Wolfe F, Kleinheksel SM, et al: Socioeconomic impact of fibrositis: a study of 81 patients with primary fibrositis. Am J Med 81 (suppl 3A):57–59, 1986

Chen M: The epidemiology of self-perceived fatigue among adults. Prev Med 15:74–81, 1986

Clark S, Campbell SM, Forehand ME, et al: Clinical characteristics of fibrositis, II: a "blinded," controlled study using standard psychological tests. Arthritis Rheum 28:132–137, 1985

Clouse RE: Anxiety and gastrointestinal illness. Psychiatr Clin North Am 11:399–417, 1988

Craig TKJ, Brown GW: Goal frustration and life events in the aetiology of painful gastrointestinal disorder. J Psychosom Res 28:411–421, 1984

Creed F, Craig T, Farmer R: Functional abdominal pain, psychiatric illness, and life events. Gut 29:235–242, 1988

Drossman DA, Powell DW, Sessions JT Jr: The irritable bowel syndrome. Gastroenterology 73:811–817, 1977

Drossman DA, McKee DC, Sandler RS, et al: Psychosocial factors in the irritable bowel syndrome: a multivariate study of patients and non-patients with irritable bowel syndrome. Gastroenterology 95:701–708, 1988

Eaton WW, Ritter C: Distinguishing anxiety and depression with field survey data. Psychol Med 18:155–166, 1988

Escobar JI: Cross-cultural aspects of the somatization trait. Hosp Community Psychiatry 38:174–180, 1987

Escobar JI, Rubio-Stipec M, Canino G, et al: Somatic Symptom Index (SSI): a new and abridged somatization construct: prevalence and epidemiological correlates in two large community samples. J Nerv Ment Dis 177:140–146, 1989

Ethington CA: The robustness of LISREL estimates in structural equation models with categorical variables. Journal of Experimental Education 55:80–88, 1987

Folgering H, Snik A: Hyperventilation syndrome and muscle fatigue. J Psychosom Res 32:165–171, 1988

Ford MJ, Miller PM, Eastwood J, et al: Life events, psychiatric illness and the irritable bowel syndrome. Gut 28:160–165, 1987

Gerster J-C, Hadj-Djilani A: Hearing and vestibular abnormalities in primary fibrositis syndrome. J Rheumatol 11:678–680, 1984

Goldenberg DL: Psychologic studies in fibrositis. Am J Med 81 (suppl 3A):67–72, 1986

Goldenberg DL: Fibromyalgia syndrome: an emerging but controversial condition. JAMA 257:2782–2787, 1987

Goldenberg DL: Research in fibromyalgia: past, present and future. J Rheumatol 15:992–996, 1988

Greenberg DB: Neurasthenia in the 1980s: chronic mononucleosis, chronic fatigue syndrome, and anxiety and depressive disorders. Psychosomatics 31:129–137, 1990

Hall W, Morrow L: "Repetition strain injury": an Australian epidemic of upper limb pain. Soc Sci Med 27:645–649, 1988

Hawley DJ, Wolfe F, Cathey MA: Pain, functional disability, and psychological status: a 12-month study of severity in fibromyalgia. J Rheumatol 15:1551–1556, 1988

Hislop IG: Psychological significance of the irritable colon syndrome. Gut 12:452–457, 1971

Holmes GP, Kaplan JE, Stewart JA, et al: A cluster of patients with a chronic mononucleosis-like syndrome. JAMA 257:2297–2302, 1987

Holmes GP, Kaplan JE, Gantz NM, et al: Chronic fatigue syndrome: a working case definition. Ann Intern Med 108:387–389, 1988

Hudson JI, Hudson MS, Pliner LF, et al: Fibromyalgia and major affective disorder: a controlled phenomenology and family history study. Am J Psychiatry 142:441–446, 1985

Jensen J: Life events in neurological patients with headache and low back pain (in relation to diagnosis and persistence of pain). Pain 32:47–53, 1988

Kellner R: Functional somatic symptoms and hypochondriasis: a survey of empirical studies. Arch Gen Psychiatry 42:821–833, 1985

Kennedy HG: Fatigue and fatiguability. Br J Psychiatry 153:1–5, 1988

Kirmayer LJ, Robbins JM, Kapusta MA: Somatization and depression in fibromyalgia syndrome. Am J Psychiatry 145:950–954, 1988

Kleinman A: Social Origins of Distress and Disease. New Haven, CT, Yale University Press, 1986

Kroenk K, Wood D, Mangelsdorff D, et al: Chronic fatigue in primary care: prevalence, patient characteristics and outcome. JAMA 260:929–934, 1988

Kruesi MJP, Dale J, Straus SE: Psychiatric diagnoses in patients who have chronic fatigue syndrome. J Clin Psychiatry 50:53–56, 1989

Kruis W, Thieme CH, Weinzierl M, et al: A diagnostic score for the irritable bowel syndrome: its value in the exclusion of organic disease. Gastroenterology 87:1–7, 1984

Kumar D, Wingate DL: The irritable bowel syndrome: a paroxysmal motor disorder. Lancet 2:973–977, 1985

Latimer P: Functional Gastrointestinal Disorders: A Behavioral Medicine Approach. New York, Springer, 1983

Liss JL, Alpers D, Woodruff RA: The irritable colon syndrome and psychiatric illness. Diseases of the Nervous System 34:151–157, 1973

Lloyd AR, Wakefield D, Boughton C, et al: What is myalgic encephalomyelitis? Lancet 1:1286–1287, 1988

Long JS: Confirmatory Factor Analysis. Beverly Hills, CA, Sage, 1983

Lowman BC, Drossman DA, Cramer EM, et al: Recollection of childhood events in adults with irritable bowel syndrome. J Clin Gastroenterology 9:324–330, 1987

Manning AP, Thompson WG, Heaton KW, et al: Towards positive diagnosis of the irritable bowel. Br Med J 2:653–654, 1978

Manu P, Lane TJ, Matthew DA: The frequency of the chronic fatigue syndrome in patients with symptoms of persistent fatigue. Ann Intern Med 109:554–556, 1988

Manu P, Lane TJ, Matthews DA: Somatization disorder in patients with chronic fatigue. Psychosomatics 30:388–395, 1989

Mayou R: Atypical chest pain. J Psychosom Res 33:393–406, 1989

McCain GA, Scudds RA: The concept of primary fibromyalgia (fibrositis): clinical value, relation and significance to other chronic musculoskeletal pain syndromes. Pain 33:273–287, 1988

McDonald EM, Mann AH, Thomas HC: Interferon as mediators of psychiatric morbidity. Lancet 2:1175–1177, 1987

Miller MH, Topliss DJ: Chronic upper limb pain syndrome (Repetitive Strain Injury) in the Australian workforce: a systematic cross sectional rheumatological study of 229 patients. J Rheumatol 15:1705–1712, 1988

Moldofsky H, Scarisbrick P, England R, et al: Musculoskeletal symptoms and non-REM sleep disturbances in patients with fibrositis syndrome and healthy subjects. Psychosom Med 37:341–351, 1975

Moldofsky H, Scarisbrick P, England R, et al: Induction of neurasthenic musculoskeletal pain syndrome by selective sleep stage deprivation. Psychosom Med 38:35–44, 1976

Moldofsky H, Tullis C, Lue FA, et al: Sleep-related myoclonus in rheumatic pain modulation disorder (fibrositis syndrome) and in excessive daytime somnolence. Psychosom Med 46:145–151, 1984

Muthen B: A general structural equation model with dichotomous, ordered categorical, and continuous latent variable indicators. Psychometrika 49:115–132, 1984

National Center for Health Statistics: The National Ambulatory Medical Care Survey: 1975 Summary. Hyattsville, MD, National Center for Health Statistics, 1978

Oettlé GJ, Heaton KW: Is there a relationship between symptoms of the irritable bowel syndrome and objective measurements of large bowel function? A longitudinal study. Gut 28:146–149, 1986

Payne TC, Leavitt F, Garron DC, et al: Fibrositis and psychologic disturbance. Arthritis Rheum 25:213–217, 1982

Pincus T, Callahan LF, Bradley LA, et al: Elevated MMPI scores for hypochondriasis, depression, and hysteria in patients with rheumatoid arthritis reflect disease rather than psychological status. Arthritis Rheum 29:1456–1466, 1986

Raskin M, Talbott JA, Meyerson AT: Diagnosis of conversion reactions: predictive value of psychiatric criteria. JAMA 197:102–106, 1966

Read N: Functional gastroenterological disorders. Gut 28:1–4, 1987

Robbins JM, Kirmayer LJ, Tepper S: Latent variable models of somatic distress. Working Papers in Social Behavior. Montreal, Department of Sociology, McGill University, No 90-1, 1990a

Robbins JM, Kirmayer LJ, Kapusta MA: Illness worry and disability in fibromyalgia syndrome. Int J Psychiatry Med 20:49–63, 1990b

Roberts RE, Vernon SW: The Center for Epidemiologic Studies Depression scale: its use in a community sample. Am J Psychiatry 140:41–46, 1983

Robins LN, Helzer JE, Croughan J, et al: National Institute of Mental Health Diagnostic Interview Schedule: its history, characteristics, and validity. Arch Gen Psychiatry 38:381–389, 1981

Robinson DP, Greene JW, Walker LS: Functional somatic complaints in adolescents: relationship to life events, self-concept, and family characteristics. J Pediatr 113:588–593, 1988

Roll M, Theorell T: Acute chest pain without obvious organic cause before age 40—personality and recent life events. J Psychosom Res 31:215–221, 1987

Sammons MT, Karoly P: Psychosocial variables in irritable bowel syndrome: a review and proposal. Clinical Psychology Review 7:187–204, 1987

Sandler RS: Epidemiology of irritable bowel syndrome in the United States. Gastroenterology 99:409–415, 1990

Sandler RS, Drossman DA, Nathan HP, et al: Symptom complaints and health care seeking behavior in subjects with bowel dysfunction. Gastroenterology 87:314–318, 1984

Scaloubaca D, Slade P, Creed F: Life events and somatisation among students. J Psychosom Res 22:221–229, 1988

Scudds RA, Rollman GB, Harth M, et al: Pain perception and personality measures as discriminators in the classification of fibrositis. J Rheumatol 14:563–569, 1987

Simon GE, Katon WJ, Sparks PJ: Allergic to life: psychological factors in environmental illness. Am J Psychiatry 147:901–908, 1990

Smith RC, Greenbaum DS, Vancouver JB, et al: Psychosocial factors are associated with health care seeking rather than diagnosis in irritable bowel syndrome. Gastroenterology 98:293–301, 1990

Smythe HA: Fibrositis and other diffuse musculoskeletal syndromes, in Textbook of Rheumatology. Edited by Kelley WN, Harris ED Jr, Ruddy S, et al. Philadelphia, PA, Saunders, 1980, pp 485–493

Stewart DE: The changing faces of somatization. Psychosomatics 31:153–158, 1990

Stewart DE, Raskin J: Psychiatric assessment of patients with "20th century disease" ("total allergy syndrome"). Can Med Assoc J 133:1001–1006, 1985

Straus SE: The chronic mononucleosis syndrome. J Infect Dis 157:405–412, 1988

Swartz M, Blazer D, Woodbury M, et al: Somatization disorder in a U.S.

Southern community: use of a new procedure for analysis of medical classification. Psychol Med 16:595–609, 1986

Taerk K, Toner B, Salit I, et al: Depression in patients with neuromyasthenia (benign encephalomyelitis). Int J Psychiatry Med 17:49–56, 1987

Talley NJ, Phillips SF, Melton LJ, et al: Diagnostic value of the Manning criteria in irritable bowel syndrome. Gut 31:77–81, 1990

Thompson WG, Heaton KW: Functional bowel disorders in apparently healthy people. Gastroenterology 79:283–288, 1980

Thompson WG, Dotevall G, Drossman DA, et al: Irritable bowel syndrome: guidelines for the diagnosis. Gastroenterology International 2:92–95, 1989

Tobi M, Straus SE: Chronic Epstein-Barr virus disease: a workshop held by the National Institute of Allergy and Infectious Disease. Ann Intern Med 103:951–953, 1985

Toner BB, Garfinkel PE, Jeejeebhoy KN, et al: Self-schema in irritable bowel syndrome and depression. Psychosom Med 52:149–155, 1990

Walker EA, Roy-Byrne PP, Katon WJ: Irritable bowel syndrome and psychiatric illness. Am J Psychiatry 147:365–372, 1990

Welch GW, Hillman LC, Pomare EW: Psychoneurotic symptomatology in the irritable bowel syndrome: a study of reporters and non-reporters. Br Med J 291:1382–1384, 1985

Welgan P, Meshkinpour H, Hoehler F: The effect of stress on colon motor and electrical activity in irritable bowel syndrome. Psychosom Med 47:139–149, 1985

Wessely S: Old wine in new bottles: neurasthenia and "ME." Psychol Med 20:35–53, 1990a

Wessely S: Chronic fatigue and myalgia syndromes, in Psychological Disorders in General Medical Settings. Edited by Sartorius N, Goldberg D, de Girolamo G, et al. Toronto, Hogrefe & Huber, 1990b, pp 82–97

Wessely S, Powell R: Fatigue syndromes: a comparison of chronic "postviral" fatigue with neuromuscular and affective disorders. J Neurol Neurosurg Psychiatry 52:940–948, 1989

Whitehead WE, Engel BT, Schuster MM: Irritable bowel syndrome: physiological and psychological differences between diarrhoea-predominant and constipation-predominant patients. Dig Dis Sci 25:404–413, 1980

Whitehead WE, Winget C, Fedoravicus AS, et al: Learned illness behavior in patients with irritable bowel syndrome and peptic ulcer. Dig Dis Sci 27:202–208, 1982

Whitehead WE, Bosmajian L, Zonderman AB, et al: Symptoms of psychologic distress associated with irritable bowel syndrome. Gastroenterology 95:709–714, 1988

Whitehead WE, Crowell MD, Bosmajian L, et al: Existence of irritable bowel syndrome supported by factor analysis of symptoms in two community samples. Gastroenterology 98:336–340, 1990

Wolfe F, Cathey MA: Prevalence of primary and secondary fibrositis. J Rheumatol 10:965–968, 1983

Wolfe F, Cathey MA: The epidemiology of tender points: a prospective study of 1520 patients. J Rheumatol 12:1164–1168, 1985

Wolfe F, Cathey MA, Kleinheksel SM, et al: Psychological status in primary fibrositis and fibrositis associated with rheumatoid arthritis. J Rheumatol 11:500–506, 1984

Wolfe F, Smythe HA, Yunus MB, et al: The American College of Rheumatology 1990 criteria for the classification of fibromyalgia: report of the Multicenter Criteria Committee. Arthritis Rheum 33:160–172, 1990

Young SJ, Alpers DH, Norland CC, et al: Psychiatric illness and the irritable bowel syndrome. Gastroenterology 70:162–166, 1976

Yunus M, Masi AT, Calabro JJ, et al: Primary fibromyalgia (fibrositis): clinical study of 50 patients with matched normal controls. Semin Arthritis Rheum 11:151–171, 1981

Zuckerman B, Stevenson J, Bailey V: Stomachaches and headaches in a community sample of preschool children. Pediatrics 79:677–682, 1987

Chapter 6

Cognitive and Social Factors in Somatization

James M. Robbins, Ph.D.,
Laurence J. Kirmayer, M.D., F.R.C.P.(C)

T he concept of somatization is relevant to our understanding of individual and cultural variations in the expression of distress, determinants of the utilization of health care resources, the success of the doctor-patient relationship, and the recognition and appropriate treatment of psychiatric disorders and psychosocial distress (Katon et al. 1982; Kleinman 1986; Lipowski 1988). Somatization has been implicated as a primary factor in work-related disability and credited with much of the hidden psychiatric morbidity in primary care (Escobar et al. 1987b; Katon et al. 1984a).

Existing research has approached the concept of somatization in three distinct ways. In the tradition of descriptive psychiatric epidemiology, somatization refers to a count of the number of medically unexplained or functional somatic symptoms during one's lifetime. In the introduction to this volume (see Chapter 1), we have called this *functional somatization*. In the study of clinical illness behavior, somatization refers to the worry or belief that one has or is vulnerable to a serious illness despite reassurances from physicians and the absence of demonstrable disease. We have called this form *hypochondriacal somatization*. In the tradition of studies of mental disorders in primary care, somatization refers to the presentation of exclusively somatic symptoms to the general practitioner despite the presence of psychiatric illness. We have called this last form *presenting somatization*.

Although acknowledged by most authors, these distinctions among forms of somatization have rarely been systematically investigated and

Preparation of this chapter was aided by a grant from the Conseil québecois de la recherche sociale. We thank Drs. Michael Dworkind and Mark Yaffe for their collaboration on this project, and Ruth Nabi for her coordination of the interview team.

107

tend to become blurred in research studies and clinical practice. In an extensive review, Kellner (1985) notes that functional somatic symptoms and hypochondriacal preoccupations, though often included together in studies, are different phenomena. Katon and colleagues (1984a) refer to two forms of somatization: 1) the presentation of physical symptoms in the absence of organic pathology and 2) the amplification of physical complaints of disease beyond what can be accounted for by physiology. Lipowski (1988) considers hypochondriasis to be a dimension within somatization along which patients may vary in their preoccupation with health and symptoms. Goldberg and Bridges (1988), reviewing somatic presentations of psychiatric illness in primary care, distinguish between patients with a history of unexplained somatic symptoms, whom the authors call "chronic somatizers," and those with a current psychiatric disorder who present to the doctor exclusively with somatic complaints. Goldberg and Bridges call the latter group of patients "subacute somatizers" and caution that they should be studied separately from chronic somatizers.

That somatization is used to refer to distinctly different phenomena by different researchers is, in itself, not a problem. Difficulties arise only when authors referring to one form of somatization make unwarranted assumptions that characteristics of that form apply equally to others. Katon and colleagues (1984b), for example, group together patients with somatic presentations of depression, somatoform disorders, and hypochondriasis, implying that they are similar clinical groups. Escobar (1987) concludes that the terms "somatization" and "hypochondriasis" refer to the same phenomenon: the presence of and preoccupation with physical symptoms. Conceptualizing somatization in this way ignores the possibility that one can be preoccupied with illness in the absence of symptoms. Attempts at more encompassing definitions of somatization also reveal fundamental equivocations. For example, Lipowski (1988) defines somatization as the tendency to experience and communicate somatic distress in response to psychosocial stress, thereby making explicit the psychological origin of somatic complaints. Elsewhere in the same article he describes somatizing patients as those who complain of physical symptoms lacking organic basis, thereby deferring the question of psychological etiology. By sharply distinguishing the different approaches in somatization research, we hope to clarify the concept and better understand the processes involved in conceptually distinct forms of somatization.

In this chapter we review the cognitive and social processes proposed to account for three forms of somatization and present evidence of the sociodemographic, psychological, and illness behavior characteristics of individuals identified by each definition. We also present original data on family medicine patients to further describe the cognitive and social similarities and differences among functional, hypochondriacal, and presenting somatizers.

A PROSPECTIVE STUDY OF SOMATIZATION IN PRIMARY CARE

The original data we present in this chapter are drawn from a study of patients attending two general hospital family medicine clinics in Montreal. Consecutive patients between the ages of 18 and 75, able to speak and read English or French and attending the clinic on a self-initiated visit or a visit for a new problem, were asked to participate. Of 1,366 potential subjects who met inclusion criteria, 698 (51%) agreed to participate and completed all measures. Thirteen patients were later excluded from the analysis because of a diagnosis of schizophrenia or organic brain syndrome, leaving 685 for whom results are presented below. Sociodemographic characteristics of the sample were comparable to those of the clinic population as a whole. The mean age was 44.4 years (SD = 16.6), and the mean number of years of education was 12.5 (SD = 4.0). Average yearly household income was Can. $24,423. Fifty-eight percent of the study subjects were female compared with 55% of all patients eligible for inclusion. Fifty percent of the sample subjects were currently married.

At the time of their visit to the clinic, patients were interviewed about their presenting complaints, current somatic and depressive symptomatology, and perceptions and beliefs about their body and health. Also, psychiatric diagnoses were made with Version III-A of the Diagnostic Interview Schedule (DIS)—a structured psychiatric interview for making DSM-III diagnoses that can be administered by trained lay interviewers (Robins et al. 1981).

One year after the their initial interview, all traceable subjects who agreed were reinterviewed about the new symptoms they had experienced over the preceding 12 months, whether those symptoms required a physician visit, the diagnoses given if any, current somatic and depressive symptomatology, and the use of mental health professionals. Of 685 patients eligible for the second interview, we were able to trace 637. Of those, complete data were obtained for 514 (80.1%). Demographic characteristics of the excluded patients were similar to those of the sample.

COGNITIVE AND SOCIAL PROCESSES IN SOMATIZATION

There has been much interest in the past decade in factors associated with the perception and appraisal of bodily symptoms. According to this cognitive-perceptual approach, bodily sensations generated by normal and abnormal processes are differentially attended to, worried about, or amplified to give rise to illness experience and behavior. Somatization, in its various forms, may then be explained as the outcome of exaggerated processes of bodily awareness, symptom preoccupation, and symptom attribution (Barsky and Klerman 1983; Kirmayer 1984, 1986). In previous work we have attempted to develop an empirical approach to examining the role of these cognitive factors in illness behavior and somatization (Robbins and Kirmayer 1986). Building on existing theories of the psychology of somatic symptoms, we have identified and simultaneously measured multiple aspects of the process of symptom perception and appraisal in clinical and epidemiologic contexts. These processes are most conveniently presented as stages in symptom experience and expression (see Figure 6-1). In reality, of course, feedback and feedforward loops knit these processes into an interactive whole that defies any simple sequential analysis (Kirmayer 1986). Nevertheless, with process-oriented longitudinal studies, it may eventually become possible to examine the temporal unfolding of illness experience and behavior.

In the following sections we outline the psychological factors that have been used by us and others to explain forms of somatization and describe the measures of these factors employed in our study of family medicine patients.

Origins of Sensations

Somatic symptoms are obvious consequences of serious organic disease and are also a prominent part of major mood and anxiety disorders (Hamilton 1989; Katon et al. 1987; Mathew et al. 1979). Yet, bodily sensations are more often generated by normal processes and minor pathological events. Physiological changes associated with digestion, respiration, exhaustion, and hormonal variation result in both specific and diffuse bodily reactions (Cannon 1929/1963). Minor symptoms associated with benign conditions like tension headache, abdominal cramps, or dyspepsia may be amplified by bodily attention and preoccupation (Barsky et al. 1988b). Bodily changes regularly accompany emotions and motivational states (Cannon 1929/1963; Grings and Dawson 1978; Schwartz et al. 1978; Shields

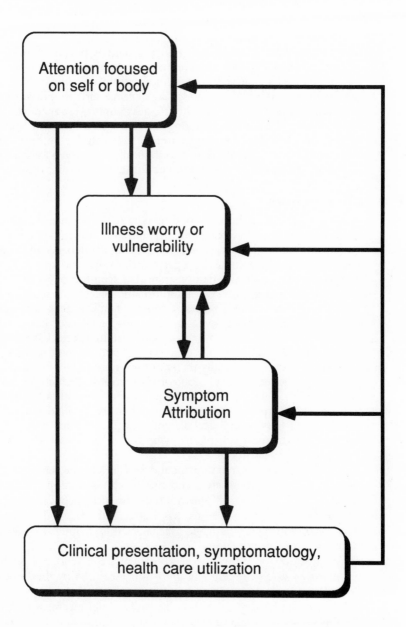

Figure 6-1. A model of cognitive processes in illness behavior.

1984). Increased autonomic nervous system activity, increased tension in voluntary muscles, and endocrine activity during emotional arousal may produce somatic symptoms in the absence of disease or structural damage. Each of these sources may produce somatic stimuli and bodily states that take on added significance and result in medical help seeking and morbidity when focused upon, exaggerated, or attributed to disease. The continuous presence of shifting bodily sensations provides the raw material that can be perceptually amplified, affectively colored, and symbolically interpreted to give rise to somatic symptoms that communicate distress of diverse origins.

Perception and Attention

Attention focused on the self or body heightens the salience of internal information and thus increases the perception of somatic symptoms. Pennebaker and colleagues (Pennebaker 1982; Pennebaker and Watson, Chapter 2, this volume) have performed a variety of experimental and naturalistic studies to demonstrate that symptom reporting increases when internal, self-relevant information exceeds that available from the environment. Joggers running a familiar track with few distractions report more somatic symptoms of fatigue than those running a novel course over complex terrain (Pennebaker and Lightner 1980). Experimental subjects instructed to attend to disruption and blockage of air flow through their nose report more nasal symptoms than those given control instructions (Pennebaker and Skelton 1978). Kellner (1985) has reviewed additional studies of mine workers who overreport chest symptoms when preoccupied with their health and of hypochondriacal patients who, more often than non-hypochondriacal subjects, report symptoms of a disease they had simply heard or read about.

People also show stable individual differences in the tendency to focus attention on themselves and their bodily sensations. Higher levels of both private self-consciousness or introspectiveness and private body-consciousness are associated with elevated somatic symptom reporting (Hansell and Mechanic 1986; Pennebaker 1982; Robbins and Kirmayer 1986).

In our study of family medicine patients, the tendency to be persistently aware of bodily sensations was measured by the Private Body-Consciousness (PBC) scale (Miller et al. 1981). The tendency to be introspectively aware of thoughts and feelings was measured by the Private Self-Consciousness (PSC) scale (Fenigstein et al. 1975). In an earlier study we found that items of the published PBC scale correlated poorly with each other (Robbins and Kirmayer 1986). To improve the reliability of the scale, we constructed three additional items, resulting in an acceptable internal consistency (alpha = .66).

Perceptual sensitivity to the environment and the body has been studied as an additional contribution to somatization. Barsky et al. (1988b) used the term *somatosensory amplification* to refer to the tendency to experience somatic sensations as intense, noxious, or disturbing. They suggested that the concept might be useful in the study of functional symptoms and variability in responding to organic disease, as well as specific functional disorders such as irritable bowel syndrome and fibromyalgia. In their study of 115 outpatients with upper respiratory tract infections, the somatosensory amplification scale was correlated at .33 with a somatic symptom measure. The amplification scale was more strongly associated with localized symptoms of upper respiratory tract infections than with generalized, systemic symptoms. Other self-report measures of autonomic perception have been shown to be associated with levels of autonomic reactivity and the tendency to overestimate autonomic levels relative to objective measures (Mandler 1984; Pennebaker 1982).

Negative affectivity (NA), a construct thought to incorporate many of the cognitive and perceptual factors discussed in this and the next subsection, may be used to explain somatization. Trait NA refers to a stable characteristic of negative mood and self concept (Pennebaker and Watson, Chapter 2, this volume; Watson and Clark 1984). Trait NA is correlated with all measures of symptom reporting. Watson and Pennebaker (1989) suggest that individuals with high NA report more symptoms, not because they are more likely to develop bodily dysfunction, but because they are more likely to perceive the dysfunction that exists. As support for this symptom perception explanation, NA and the related construct *neuroticism* have been shown to be associated with self-focus, worry, and hypochondriacal attitudes (Costa and McCrae 1985; Watson and Clark 1984; Watson and Pennebaker 1989). Negative mood is also known to increase illness memories and contribute to a negative view of one's health (Croyle and Uretsky 1987). Some psychodynamic accounts of somatization view it as a mode of coping with feelings of guilt, anger, and low self-esteem—all of which are attributes included in the NA construct.

Our measure of NA in the family medicine study is the RD16 scale (Schuessler et al. 1978). This scale was designed as a measure of the tendency to respond in the socially desirable direction to attitude-opinion items. Although the authors argue against considering this scale an indicator of a cheerful and benign temperament, others (McCrae and Costa 1983) suggest that scales such as this are most appropriately used as measures of optimism or well-being (or inversely, neuroticism) as opposed to a responding artifact to be controlled in substantive research. NA is thus taken by us to refer to the low end of the RD16 scale.

Recognition and Interpretation

Illness worry, or hypochondriasis, is also thought to increase somatic symptomatology. Although we believe that hypochondriasis is a distinct form of somatization, it often coexists with functional somatization. The belief that one has or is vulnerable to serious illness, and the preoccupation with disease, most likely motivate vigilant scanning of the body for unusual sensations and the recognition of those sensations as symptoms of illness. Conversely, having persistent pain and somatic distress repeatedly discounted by physicians as functional can result in preoccupation with symptoms and fear of disease.

The association between hypochondriasis and somatic symptoms has been studied most often with the Whitely Index of hypochondriasis and the Illness Behavior Questionnaire (IBQ), developed by Pilowsky and colleagues (Pilowsky 1967; Pilowsky et al. 1979). The Whitely Index, a measure of hypochondriacal beliefs, has been shown to be moderately correlated with somatic symptom scales. Barsky et al. (1986) reported a .52 correlation between the Whitely Index and a scale of 12 somatic symptom items among a sample of general medical outpatients. In our earlier study of family medicine patients, a scale measuring worries about being vulnerable to a serious illness, based on the IBQ, correlated at .40 with the somatization subscale of the Symptom Checklist-90 (Robbins and Kirmayer 1986). Without ruling out physical disease that could otherwise explain the patient's illness worry, however, it is questionable whether the term *hypochondriasis* ought to be applied to the Whitely Index and scales based on it (Costa and McCrae 1985; Zonderman et al. 1985).

In our study, hypochondriacal attitude was measured by the Illness Worry Scale. This scale consists of nine items, derived from the IBQ (Pilowsky and Spence 1983), that measure the tendency for people to worry that bodily sensations or feelings signify serious disease and to feel vulnerable to falling ill. The scale has moderate internal consistency (alpha = .70).

Attribution and Help Seeking

Somatization may also result from misattribution of benign bodily sensations to serious illness (Stoeckle and Barsky 1980). Barsky and Klerman (1983) point out that somatization may arise when individuals are unable to discount sensations that most other people would attribute to fatigue, aging, dietary indiscretion, or normal physiological processes. We have constructed a scale to measure the tendency to attribute common somatic symptoms to physical illness or to psychological causes such as mood or stress, or to discount them by invoking environmental or normalizing explanations (Robbins and Kirmayer 1990). The Symptom Interpretation Questionnaire (SIQ) yields three scales representing these modes of attribution. When tested on an earlier sample of 100 family medicine patients, those scoring higher on the somatic SIQ scale presented more somatic symptoms, and more somatic symptoms of obscure origin, to the clinic when followed up for 6 months (Robbins and Kirmayer 1986, 1990). Patients scoring higher on the normalizing SIQ scale presented significantly fewer psychosocial symptoms, although no fewer somatic symptoms.

Social Factors

Cognitive and perceptual factors are often suggested as mediators of sociodemographic differences in illness behavior and somatization (Kirmayer 1984, 1986), although these explanations remain to be confirmed with representative samples such as those of the Epidemiologic Catchment Area studies (Eaton and Kessler 1985). Women, for example, are thought to be more attuned to their bodies than men and therefore more likely to recognize and report symptoms (Pennebaker and Watson, Chapter 2, this volume; Verbrugge 1985). Interestingly, when men are required to focus on their symptoms by completing a daily health diary, they report comparable numbers of illnesses (Bishop 1984). Lower socioeconomic status is thought to increase the likelihood that distress will be perceived as physical disease rather than as emotional disorder (Bart 1968; Crandell and Dohrenwend 1967). Cross-cultural differences in somatization have also been explained by cognitive and social factors (Angel and Thoits 1987; Kirmayer 1984). Higher somatization among Hispanics may be due to the greater stigma associated with mental illness among that group, the belief that emotion is an indication of weakness, and less psychological mindedness (Escobar et al. 1987a, 1989). In epidemiologic studies, nonmarried people report more somatic symptoms (Schwab et al. 1978). People living alone may be more internally focused than those cohabiting, suggesting that those individuals with fewer competing external demands notice physical symptoms more often than those with more frequent social obligations (Pennebaker 1982).

Family and social influences are also proposed as causal factors in somatization. Somatic symptoms in the family and parental attitudes toward health influence a child's focus of attention and enhance perception of somatic processes (Wilkinson 1988). Children's symptoms often resemble those of family members (Craig 1978; Turkat et al. 1984), and a child's attentiveness to symptoms is related to the mother's interest in the child's illness (Mechanic 1964). Other studies have shown that encouragement to adopt the sick role as a child is related to increased symptom reports, clinic visits, and disability days in adulthood (Pilowsky et al. 1982; Whitehead et al. 1986). Lipowski (1988) concludes that social learning is a particularly important factor predisposing one to somatize. Learning to focus on somatic sensations, interpret them as threatening, express them verbally, and use them to communicate distress occurs in the context of the family. Families may, however, resent somatization as well as reinforce it. Lennon et al. (1989) recognize the dilemma faced by patients with a history of functional symptoms who must seek treatment in order to socially validate their subjective distress but who, when treatment fails repeatedly, are seen by family and friends as personally weak or lacking the motivation to get better.

THREE FORMS OF SOMATIZATION

In this section we apply the results reviewed above and those of our own study to understand the three forms of somatization identified in the introduction to this chapter. Beginning with functional somatization, we present evidence of the prevalence and sociodemographic profile, followed by the cognitive and perceptual factors associated with this form of somatization. Hypochondriacal somatization is then considered, followed by presenting somatization. The pattern of results presented in this section is summarized in Tables 6-1 and 6-2.

Somatization as Medically Unexplained or Functional Somatic Symptoms

We use the term *functional somatization* to refer to a history of many medically unexplained somatic symptoms. This form of somatization has been studied in the context of patients presenting to specialty clinics with discrete forms of unexplained somatic distress (as reviewed by Kirmayer and Robbins, Chapter 5, this volume) and in samples of the general population as part of the National Institute of Mental Health (NIMH) Epidemiologic Catchment Area (ECA) program. Functional somatization in the community has been studied most thoroughly by Escobar, Swartz, and colleagues (see Chapter 4, this volume). In a series of studies based on the ECA program, somatization has been defined in terms of the number of medically unexplained symptoms among the 37 items included in the DIS diagnosis of somatization disorder. The total number of medically unexplained symptoms on the DIS has been termed the Somatic Symptom Index

Table 6-1. Sociodemographic characteristics of three forms of somatization

Sociodemographic characteristic	Form of somatization		
	Functional[a]	Hypochondriacal[b]	Presenting[c]
Age	+/0[d]	0	0
Female	+	0	−?
Married	−	0	0
Income	−	−	0
Working full or part time	0	−	0
Education	−	−	0
Urban resident	+	*	*
Immigrant to North America	0	+	0
Hispanic ethnicity	+	*	*

[a]Number of medically unexplained somatic symptoms on the Diagnostic Interview Schedule.
[b]Scores on the Whitely Index and/or Illness Worry Scale.
[c]Presenting somatizers compared to psychosocial presenters.
[d]Table entries indicate positive relationship with the characteristic (+), negative relationship (−), no relationship (0), or not yet studied in this context (*).

Table 6-2. Illness cognition characteristics of three forms of somatization

Illness cognition measure	Form of somatization[a]		
	Functional	Hypochondriacal	Presenting[b]
Body-consciousness	+	+	0
Self-consciousness	+	+	0
Illness worry	+/0	+ (defined)	0
Emotion worry	+	+	−
Psychological attribution	+	+	− −c
Somatic attribution	0	+	0
Normalizing attribution	−	−	+ +
Negative affectivity	+	+ +	0

[a]See Table 6-1 for definitions.
[b]Presenting somatizers compared with psychosocial presenters.
[c]Strong relationships indicated by double symbols (+ +, − −).

(SSI). In an effort to identify respondents who are more likely to be heavy users of health services, Escobar and colleagues (1989) have proposed a level of four symptoms for men and six symptoms for women (SSI 4,6) as criteria for a subsyndromal form of somatization disorder.

Prevalence and sociodemographic characteristics. Prevalence estimates of any disorder assume that the condition is an entity that is either present or absent. It is not immediately clear whether functional somatization ought to be seen as a discrete condition or better understood as a dimensional construct. Because typical measures of functional somatization are based on somewhat arbitrary cutoffs within a continuous scale from no medically unexplained symptoms during one's lifetime to 37 symptoms, prevalence estimates will vary depending on the location of the cutoff. When the SSI 4,6 criteria are used, between 9% and 20% of the general population across the five ECA sites are identified as functional somatizers (Escobar et al. 1989). When the SSI is retained in its full, continuous metric, community residents report an average of 3.2 (SD = 3.8) functional symptoms over their lifetime (Swartz et al. 1987). In our sample of 685 family medicine patients, the mean value on the SSI was 2.2 (SD = 2.6) for men and 3.8 (SD = 3.3) for women. Only 1% of patients met DSM-III criteria for somatization disorder (SSI 12,14), while 17% (n = 114) reached the SSI 4,6 criterion.

In the general population, medically unexplained symptoms are more likely to occur among women, those who are not married, those with less education and income, nonwhites, Hispanics, older subjects, and urban residents (Escobar 1987; Escobar et al. 1987a, 1989; Swartz et al. 1986a, 1987, 1988, 1989). These relationships are summarized in the first column of Table 6-1.

In our study of family medicine patients, women, unmarried persons, and those with less education and income reported more medically unexplained symptoms. Contrary to studies of the general population, older patients reported no more unexplained symptoms than did younger patients (see Table 6-1). Although the sociodemographic relationships among our clinic-based sample are very similar to those of community-based samples, these findings as well as others we will report below are likely influenced by factors affecting self-selection into care among our subjects.

Psychological determinants. Studies of functional somatization based on samples of the general population have not yet focused on processes of perception, cognition, or attribution as predictors of medically unexplained symptoms. Findings do exist, however, for general clinic-based samples and samples of patients selected for specific medically unexplained somatic syndromes.

In our study, medically unexplained symptoms were found to be significantly, though very weakly, correlated with attention focused toward the self or body.[1] The SSI correlated at only .10 ($P = .004$) with the PSC scale and .17 ($P < .001$) with the expanded version of the PBC scale (see Table 6-2). In another study, body-consciousness failed to discriminate between patients with the functional somatic syndrome of fibromyalgia and patients with rheumatoid arthritis, a symptomatically comparable organic disease (Robbins et al. 1990).

Hypochondriacal beliefs were modestly correlated with functional symptoms among our sample. The number of functional somatic symptoms correlated at .29 ($P < .001$) with the Illness Worry Scale. When patients with current serious illness were removed from the analysis to approximate more closely hypochondriacal worry, the correlation remained significant, although still modest ($r = .28$, $P < .001$).

Although Pilowsky and Spence (1975) found that chronic pain patients score higher on illness worry measures than do family practice patients, other studies show no difference between patients with unexplained or exaggerated symptoms and patients with organic illness (Joyce et al. 1986; Kellner and Schneider-Braus 1988; Kirmayer and Robbins, Chapter 5, this volume; Robbins et al. 1990) (see Table 6-2). It is unclear, therefore, to what extent hypochondriasis may be an etiological factor in functional somatization or an outcome of persistent or recurrent physical illness with or without adequate medical explanation.

Symptom attribution may also play a role in the experience and reporting of functional somatic complaints. Aside from the brief questionnaire administered by Wessely and Powell (1989) to patients with chronic fatigue syndrome, attributions of the origin of symptoms have not previously been studied in the context of functional somatization. We administered the SIQ to our family medicine sample. Those with a greater number of medically unexplained symptoms scored significantly lower on the normalizing SIQ ($r = -.20$, $P < .001$), indicating that they were less likely to discount

---

[1]Although we report bivariate relationships in this chapter, these have been verified in multivariate models. The correlations we report are taken from panels of 26 sociodemographic, illness cognition, and illness behavior variables for each form of somatization. Multiple tests increase the risk of a Type I error. With a sample size of 685, a correlation of $r \geq .11$ will maintain an overall Type I error rate of .05.

common symptoms by attributing them to environmental events. These individuals also scored higher on the psychological SIQ ($r = .20$, $P < .001$), suggesting a tendency to attribute common somatic symptoms to mood or stress. There was no correlation between the somatic SIQ and the number of functional symptoms (see Table 6-2). Thus, patients with more functional symptoms are more likely to choose a pathological explanation for somatic symptoms but do not display an overall bias toward attributing common symptoms to physical illness.

Somatization as Hypochondriacal Worry

Hypochondriacal somatization is taken by us to refer to the tendency to worry about the possibility that one has or is vulnerable to a serious physical illness. While this form of somatization is generally recognized as distinct from functional somatization, for some authors, illness preoccupation and symptom experience are so intertwined as to be indistinguishable (Mabe et al. 1988; Swartz et al. 1986b). Yet, even for those authors who confound functional and hypochondriacal somatization, hypochondriasis is most often gauged by self-report scales—such as the Whitely Index, the Health Worry Scale (Zonderman et al. 1985), or the Illness Attitudes Scales (Kellner 1987)—that measure predominately worry or attitudinal preoccupation with illness, not symptom or disease experience (Barsky et al. 1986).

Prevalence and sociodemographic characteristics. The prevalence of hypochondriacal somatization is difficult to estimate because of variability in definitions and diagnostic criteria. Because many measures are based on continuous scales, the distinction between hypochondriacal somatizers and nonsomatizers is often only a matter of degree. Summarizing existing studies, Kellner (1985) reported that rates of hypochondriasis range from 3% to 13% of the population and that illness worries, varying from rational concerns to constant, incapacitating fears, occur in 10%. In his own study of family practice patients, Kellner and colleagues (1983) found that 9% refused to believe the physician's reassurance that they did not have a serious illness. This finding conforms closely to our estimate of 8% for the prevalence of hypochondriasis in 685 family medicine patients based on high scores on the Illness Worry Scale and low scores on a rating of seriousness of concurrent medical disease (Kirmayer and Robbins, in press).

Literature on the social worlds and social characteristics of hypochondriacal somatizers is inconsistent. For example, the stereotype of older people as more hypochondriacal appears to be confirmed by studies of symptom reports, physician utilization, and scores on the Minnesota Multiphasic Personality Inventory (MMPI) hypochondriasis scale. Yet, each of these outcomes is influenced as much by physical illness, which increases with age, as by exaggerated illness worry (Costa and McCrae 1985). Physical illness must be ruled out before measures of illness behavior and illness worry can be presumed to indicate hypochondriasis (Zonderman et al. 1985). Age was unrelated to illness worry in our study of patients ($r = -.02$).

In contrast to functional somatization, which is more prevalent among women, men are sometimes found to score higher on measures of illness worry and disease conviction (Pilowsky et al. 1987). In other well-designed studies using the Whitely Index and the IBQ, however, no sex differences have been observed (Barsky and Wyshak 1989; Barsky et al. 1986; Zonderman et al. 1985). Men and women received identical scores on our Illness Worry Scale. Also in contrast to functional somatization, which appears to be more common among those with lower education and income, social position has usually been found to be unrelated to scores on the Whitely Index, although the power to detect such associations in these studies has been quite limited (Barsky and Wyshak 1989; Barsky et al. 1986). In our study, with greater statistical power, high scores on illness worry were significantly—although only slightly—more likely among those with lower education ($r = -.20$, $P < .001$), those with lower income ($r = -.19$, $P < .001$), those not in the labor force ($r = -.08$, $P = .02$), and immigrants to North America ($r = -.11$, $P = .002$). Barsky and colleagues (1986) found no marital status differences on the Whitely Index among their sample of medical outpatients, a finding replicated on the Illness Worry Scale with our sample. Relationships between hypochondriacal somatization and sociodemographic characteristics are summarized in the second column of Table 6-1.

A social-learning explanation has been proposed in a number of theoretical models of hypochondriacal somatization (Barsky et al. 1986; Kellner 1985), but we have been able to locate only one study that addresses this thesis directly. Mabe and colleagues (1988) tested whether learned social behaviors might be predictive of scores on their hypochondriacal index. This composite measure consisted of the Whitely Index, the patient's overestimation of the severity of his or her illness compared to the physician's estimation, and physicians' ratings of whether the patient's illness presentation exceeded demonstrable disease. When tested on 100 general medical inpatients, past serious illness and acceptance of illness as part of life significantly predicted hypochondriasis. Notably, the belief that parents were attentive when the patient was sick as a child was not related to the patient's score on the outcome index.

Hypochondriacal beliefs in our sample were more likely to occur among those who spoke more frequently to a significant other about their health ($r = .25$, $P < .001$) and who felt that their significant other worried more about the possibility that the patient had a serious illness ($r = .40$, $P < .001$). Thus, there is some support for hypochondriacal somatization as a consequence of social validation of distress. Correlational findings, however, cannot rule out the likelihood that somatizers simply bring their complaints home for discussion.

Psychological determinants. Cognitive and perceptual processes similar to those offered to explain functional somatization may be involved in hypochondriacal somatization as well. Barsky and colleagues (1988a) have offered just such a model of hypochondriasis and have tailored a treatment approach to their theoretical assumptions. According to their view, worry about the possibility that one has a serious illness begins with cognitive and perceptual deficits that cause a person to experience normal bodily sensations as particularly noxious and intense. Hypochondriacal beliefs including mistrust of doctors, resistance to reassurance, bodily preoccupation, and disease conviction are seen as secondary to sensory amplification. There is evidence to support the assumption that hypochondriacal individuals may be more sensitive to sensory stimuli (Hanback and Revelle 1978), have less tolerance for experimental pain (Ziesat 1978), and exhibit lower pain thresholds than other individuals (Merskey and Evans 1975). The model of Barsky and colleagues (1988a), however, hinges on the additional assumption that because sensations are experienced as so disturbing, hypochondriacal individuals mistakenly attribute these sensations to serious disease and conclude that they are ill.

A number of studies, including our own, indicate that attributions of sensations to pathological processes can increase symptoms (Robbins and Kirmayer 1990; Rodin 1978). But these studies do not confirm that misattributions necessarily arise because sensations are experienced as particularly disturbing. It is equally likely that attributions of new sensations to serious illness are based on cognitive schemas established by prior episodes of illness. Experiencing a serious illness probably provides a ready schema for interpreting new bodily sensations while increasing one's vigilance toward future illness. New sensations may thus be seen as more threatening, more distressing, and as confirming evidence of a new illness because they fit existing illness schemas, not because of cognitive and perceptual deficits.

Illness need not be organic for a person to become preoccupied with the possibility of disease. As Lennon and colleagues (1989) suggest, the prolonged search for social validation of functional symptoms may lead to preoccupation with the condition and its cause. Many people with undeniable subjective distress, in addition to seeking symptomatic relief, seek to convince others that the distress is real. Some may be required by disability boards to provide medical verification of illness. Some may seek verification as a sign to others that they wish to be well. For distress to become a social reality, sufferers must receive validation from a physician. Yet, because functional symptoms do not fit a standard biomedical explanatory scheme, social validation is often not forthcoming. As a result, patients may become preoccupied with their illness and with the search for the one explanation that will convince others of the reality of their discomfort and incapacitation. The more they are investigated, the more they become convinced that there is a hidden physical illness. The resistance of hypochondriacal patients to reassurance and these patients' ultimate mistrust of physicians may be partly understood in the context of these social pressures.

Hypochondriacal somatization often accompanies psychiatric disorders, including depression, anxiety, obsessive-compulsive disorder, schizophrenia, and personality disorders (Kenyon 1976). Barsky et al. (1986) found that 27% of a sample of medical outpatients who scored high on the Whitely Index had major psychiatric diagnoses recorded in their medical charts compared with only 3% of those who scored low on the index. In our study, 36% of patients meeting criteria for only hypochondriacal somatization had a lifetime diagnosis of major depression or anxiety compared with 21% of nonsomatizers. Of those meeting criteria for both functional (4 or above on a count of medically unexplained symptoms) and hypochondriacal somatization, 49% were diagnosed with psychiatric disorders ($\chi^2(3) = 42.9$, $P < .001$).

Many studies have demonstrated a substantial relationship between measures of depressive symptomatology and hypochondriasis (Fava et al. 1982; Mabe et al. 1988). In Barsky's study of medical outpatients, the Beck Depression Inventory was correlated at .56 with the Whitely Index (Barsky et al. 1986). Zonderman et al. (1985) found a correlation of about .5 between IBQ-derived scales of health worry and affective disturbance in their sample of over 1,000 subjects. In our study, the correlation between the Center for Epidemiologic Studies Depression (CES-D) scale (Radloff 1977) and illness worry was .43 ($P < .001$). Mabe and colleagues (1988) have offered four explanations of why affective disturbance should be related to hypochondriasis:

1. Distress may precipitate hypochondriasis by producing physiological changes that can be construed as disease.
2. Distress may lead to intolerance of discomfort and preoccupation with symptoms previously ignored.
3. Hypochondriasis may cause emotional distress if symptoms are not taken seriously by the physician.
4. Distress and hypochondriasis may both be related to the underlying personality dimension of neuroticism or NA.

Like Mabe and coworkers (1988), Pennebaker and Watson (Chapter 2, this volume) suggest that NA may be a latent variable that causes both functional symptom reporting and hypochondriasis. Our data support the role of NA in hypochondriasis but less so in functional somatization. Pure hypochondriacal somatizers (i.e., those without functional symptoms) are best distinguished from pure functional somatizers (i.e., those without hypochondriacal beliefs) by their negative, pessimistic, foreboding view of themselves and the world. Whereas functional somatizers score about the same as nonsomatizers on the RD16, a measure we take to indicate a cheerful and benign temperament ($\overline{X}_{func} = 12.7$, SD = 2.6; $\overline{X}_{non} = 13.2$, SD = 2.2), hypochondriacal somatizers score much lower on this scale ($\overline{X}_{hyp} = 11.5$, SD = 2.7, $F(3, 682) = 24.4$, $P < .001$) and show a pattern indicative of a worrying, concerned cognitive style on other measures, including private self-consciousness ($F(3, 682) = 11.1$, $P < .001$), private body-consciousness ($F(3, 682) = 16.0$, $P < .001$), normalizing symptom attribution ($F(3, 682) = 16.6$, $P < .001$), and depressive symptomatology (CES-D, $F(3, 682) = 45.1$, $P < .001$) (see Table 6-2). Interestingly, functional somatizers who are not also hypochondriacal have RD16, self-consciousness, body-consciousness, and CES-D scores comparable to those of nonsomatizers. It is only when functional somatizers also have hypochondriacal beliefs that they too score high on measures of NA.

Thus, NA may have a more immediate and direct etiological connection to hypochondriasis than to functional somatization. The most appropriate specification of the association among NA, functional symptoms, and hypochondriacal beliefs remains to be determined. NA may be antecedent only to hypochondriasis, affecting symptom reporting only indirectly through its effect on illness worry and disease preoccupation. Structural models of these relationships may uncover the predominant causal effects.

Somatization as the Somatic Presentation of Psychiatric Disorder

Patients who present to health care providers complaining primarily of somatic symptoms, but who are also found to have major depression or anxiety that may account for those symptoms, are the most commonly studied examples of this third form of somatization (Bridges and Goldberg 1985; Katon et al. 1982; Kirmayer and Robbins, in press). Gradations of presenting somatization can be identified based on the degree of patients' reluctance to acknowledge a psychosocial dimension to their distress. Bridges and Goldberg (1985) distinguished between facultative and true "somatizers." While both types of patients made somatic presentations of psychiatric disorders, the former acknowledged psychological distress when skillfully interviewed, while the latter persisted in rejecting any psychological attribution for their symptoms.

Prevalence and sociodemographic characteristics. Recent detailed reviews of the prevalence of mental disorders in primary care conclude that current psychiatric disorders, most often major depression and anxiety, are present in 25% to 30% of patients who visit general practitioners (Blacker and Clare 1987; Katon 1987; Schulberg and Burns 1988). Over 50% of those individuals with diagnosable disorders—perhaps as high as 80%—present with somatic rather than psychiatric symptoms (Bridges and Goldberg 1985; Goldberg and Bridges 1988). In our study, 11% of the sample received current DIS diagnoses of major depression or anxiety disorders (primarily panic disorder). Of these patients, 21% presented with at least one psychosocial complaint. We have called this group "psychosocial presenters." Of the remaining group of somatic presenters, 29 of 55 (53%) made spontaneous psychosocial attributions when asked what they felt caused their somatic symptoms. These we term "initial somatizers." Consistent with the definitions of Bridges and Goldberg (1985), the remaining 26 patients were divided into "facultative somatizers" ($n = 17$) who, when asked directly, accepted nerves or worries as a possible cause of their somatic distress, and "true somatizers" ($n = 9$) who continued to reject nerves or worries even when asked directly. (Five additional patients were excluded from the analysis because they came to the clinic on a health maintenance visit and presented no symptoms.) In the analyses below we will compare the aggregate group of presenting somatizers with psychosocial presenters, commenting on the subgroups of somatizers where relevant.

Although there are prevailing beliefs about the social, demographic, and cultural characteristics of presenting somatizers, the few studies on this form of somatization are inconclusive. It is often stated, for example, that people from lower socioeconomic classes are more likely than those from the middle and upper socioeconomic classes to somatize psychiatric disorder. People with less education and income are felt to be less psychologically minded and, because of negative attitudes toward mental illness, more resistant to acknowledging psychological distress. Goldberg and Bridges (1988), however, in a study of 500 patients who presented new illnesses to family doctors in Manchester, found that those who somatized current psychiatric illness were from socioeconomic-class backgrounds that were comparable to those of individuals who psychologized their disorders. In our study, presenting somatizers were no different than psychosocial presenters in schooling, income, marital status, age, or labor force participation. A somewhat higher proportion of true somatizers were men (44%) compared with psychosocial presenters (30%), although the difference did not reach significance. There were no substantial marital status or immigration differences among groups (see Table 6-1).

In a parallel analysis conducted to increase the power of comparisons among groups, we replaced current DIS diagnosis with high scores on the CES-D scale as the indicator of psychiatric disorder. Of all patients, 202 (29%) scored 16 or above on the CES-D scale, a value often used in screening for cases of depression (Roberts and Vernon 1983). Using the classification scheme above, 31 of these patients (15%) were considered psychosocial presenters, 69 (34%) were initial somatizers, 52 (26%) were facultative somatizers, and 50 (25%) were true somatizers. As above, no differences were noted in any sociodemographic characteristics except sex. Sixty percent of true somatizers were men compared with 30% of facultative and initial somatizers and 40% of psychosocial presenters ($P = .003$).

Psychological determinants. Cognitive and perceptual factors have not previously been studied in the context of presenting somatization. In our study, presenting somatizers (true or facultative) could not be distinguished from psychosocial presenters on measures of self-consciousness, body-consciousness, or illness worry. All three groups, however, were distinct on a measure of emotion worry. Emotion worry was assessed by an 8-item scale (alpha = .81) designed to measure the tendency to conclude that fluctuations in feelings signify a serious emotional problem. Psychosocial presenters scored very high on this scale ($X = 4.0$, SD = 2.0), while true somatizers scored very low ($X = 1.9$, SD = 2.0) and facultative and initial somatizers were intermediate ($F(3, 198) = 8.8$, $P < .001$).

The most striking and consistent cognitive differences between somatizers and psychosocial presenters in our study were on measures of symptom attribution. The patterns of results were identical whether psychiatric disorder is defined by DIS diagnoses or by high values on the CES-D scale, although because of greater power the results for groups identified using the CES-D scale were sometimes statistically significant when the more restrictive DIS-based results were not. These results are summarized in Table 6-2. Consistent with their symptom presentation, true somatizers (i.e., presenting somatizers) scored significantly lower on the scale measuring the tendency to attribute common somatic symptoms to psychological causes ($F(3, 198) = 8.9$, $P < .001$) and significantly higher on the scale measuring the tendency to attribute symptoms to normal conditions or environmental circumstances ($F(3, 198) = 4.5$, $P = .005$). Interestingly, when compared on the Cognitive Somatic Anxiety Questionnaire (CSAQ) (Schwarz et al. 1978), somatizers were less likely than psychosocial presenters to report both cognitive ($F(3, 197) = 5.3$, $P < .002$) and somatic ($F(3, 194) = 3.6$, $P = .01$) symptoms in response to anxiety. Conceptually, the CSAQ is the converse of the SIQ, because it asks subjects which symptoms they tend to experience when anxious, whereas the SIQ asks whether common somatic symptoms would be attributed to anxiety or other emotional distress. These results suggest that psychosocial presenters have an underlying "psychosomatic" cognitive schema relating physical symptoms and emotional distress (Helman 1985). In contrast, somatizers acknowledge no such psychosomatic connection.

These findings are most likely not due to a difference in NA among the groups, since scores on the RD16 are virtually identical. They may, however, be related to the lack of recognition or reporting of dysphoric symptoms among true somatizers. Among groups chosen on the basis of current DIS diagnoses, confirming the presence of major depression or anxiety, true somatizers reported significantly fewer symptoms on the CES-D scale ($\overline{X} = 15.3$, SD = 10.5) than did facultative and initial somatizers ($\overline{X} = 24.1$, SD = 10.7) or psychosocial presenters ($\overline{X} = 29.3$, SD = 10.4, $F(3, 66) = 2.7$, $P = .05$). The results are similar, though not quite significant, when major depression alone is used as the criterion for psychiatric disorder. Thus, even though suffering a current major depression or anxiety disorder, presenting somatizers may not report the symptoms of dysphoria necessary for a psychosocial presentation.

The lack of acknowledgement of psychosomatic relationships and of emotional distress among presenting somatizers fits other evidence of their illness attitudes. For example, Goldberg and Bridges (1988) found that presenting somatizers had more hostile attitudes toward mental illness and would be less likely to seek help for symptoms of depression or anxiety than would psychosocial presenters.

There is no evidence that presenting somatizers have learned to model their somatic presentation from others or that their somatization constitutes provisional validation of the sick role. Goldberg and Bridges (1988) found no evidence that the memories of childhood illnesses were any different for somatizers than for psychosocial presenters. Spouses of somatizers were no more or less sympathetic when the patient was ill, and somatizers were no more or less likely to have discussed their symptoms with family members. In our study, somatizers talked to their closest friend or relative about their health no more often than did psychosocial presenters.

Presenting somatization, then, appears to be related to a consistent attributional bias that may reflect the lack of a psychosomatic schema linking emotional and somatic distress. This psychosomatic connection is not conceptually difficult to learn, so the rejection of such explanations may reflect a defensive avoidance of the frightening, stigmatizing, and socially unacceptable implications of emotional or psychiatric illness. Alternatively, rejection of such a connection may be traced to the relative salience of the physical symptoms of depression and anxiety, and/or to a heightened sensitivity to normative constraints that discourage open expression of emotion (Kirmayer 1987).

THE ILLNESS BEHAVIOR OF SOMATIZERS

The concept of somatization draws our attention to the disjunction between disease and illness. Models of somatization allow us to understand the conditions under which medically unexplained symptoms are likely to persist, when hypochondriacal beliefs will extend beyond private worry to help-seeking behavior, and how somatic presentations of psychiatric disorder arise from, and subsequently influence, the natural history of the disorder.

Somatization entails great social costs (Escobar et al. 1987b; Kellner 1985). Because diagnosis and treatment are often inconclusive, avid consumption of medical services by somatizers may lead to extensive examination and laboratory investigation (Escobar et al. 1987a). This intensive use of health care resources represents an economic burden and, if followed by inappropriate diagnosis and treatment, places the somatizer at risk for iatrogenic injury (Kellner 1985). Somatization is also held to increase personal and corporate costs through frequent sick leave and activity restriction (Smith et al. 1986).

Escobar and colleagues (1987b) have used the Los Angeles ECA data to study the health care utilization and disability of functional somatizers. When followed up after 6 months, respondents meeting the SSI 4,6 criteria were more likely than other respondents to have experienced restricted activity or to have spent at least one day in bed and to have used general medical services for mental health problems. Functional somatizers were no more likely than nonsomatizers to have used specialty mental health care.

The illness behavior of hypochondriacal somatizers has been studied by relating scores on the Whitely Index and the IBQ to number of physician visits, laboratory tests, preventive health behaviors, and no-show rates. Pilowsky et al. (1987) studied the relationship between the IBQ and utilization among 95 general practice patients. The disease conviction scale was predictive of the number of physician contacts over the following 6 months. Neither the Whitely Index nor the general hypochondriasis scale, however, predicted number of contacts. Barsky and Wyshak (1989) studied the illness behavior correlates of the Whitely Index among 177 outpatients at a general medical clinic. Number of health system contacts correlated at .31 with the Whitely Index, while self-treatments with vitamins, health foods, and other health precautions correlated at .20. Beaber and Rodney (1984), in a study of 109 family practice patients, found that those who scored high on the Whitely Index were more likely to have received screening laboratory testing and to have had high no-show rates.

Although we have taken pains to distinguish among somatization constructs, clinical and epidemiologic reality is also served by acknowledging the juxtaposition of different forms of somatization. We might expect, for example, that people who meet criteria for both functional and hypochondriacal forms of somatization will be particularly problematic. These individuals hold fast to the belief that they have a serious illness even though the pathology of their somatic distress has been repeatedly discounted by a physician. To explore how the combination of illness worry and frequent medically unexplained symptoms differs from pure groups of somatizers, we compared patients meeting criteria for both functional and hypochondriacal somatization, "pure" groups meeting criteria for only one form of somatization, and nonsomatizers on 1-year prospective health care utilization data (see Table 6-3). For this analysis, functional somatizers were those who reported a lifetime history of four or more medically unexplained symptoms ($n = 129$, 27%). Hypochondriacal somatizers were those who scored 3 or above on the Illness Worry Scale ($n = 98$, 19.1%). Patients meeting criteria for both forms (8% of the follow-up sample of 514) reported more physician visits over the ensuing year ($F(3, 510) = 5.0$, $P = .002$), more somatic symptoms that resulted in a physician visit ($F(3, 510) = 29.7$, $P < .001$), and more symptoms given no diagnosis ($F(3, 510) = 22.8$, $P < .001$) than did patients meeting criteria for either functional somatization only (19.1%) or hypochondriacal somatization only (11.1%), or non-somatizers (61.9%). They were also more likely to have been hospitalized ($\chi^2(3) = 8.5$, $P = .04$), to have visited a nonpsychiatric physician for emotional problems ($\chi^2(3) = 39.5$, $P < .001$), and to have visited a mental health professional ($\chi^2(3) = 9.7$, $P = .02$). Pure functional somatizers utilized services more than did pure hypochondriacal somatizers. Hypochondriacal somatizers were no different than nonsomatizers on most utilization measures. Thus, when followed for a year, functional somatizers continued to make

Table 6-3. Illness behavior characteristics of somatizers

Illness behavior during 12-month follow-up	Type of somatizer		
	Functional and hypochondriacal[a]	Functional only[b]	Hypochondriacal only[c]
Talked to other about health	+[d]	0	+
Number of health care visits	+ +	+	+
Hospitalized	+	0	0
Number of somatic symptoms	+	+	0
Number of somatic symptoms resulting in physician visit	+ +	+	0
Number of unexplained somatic symptoms	+ +	+	0
Number of psychological symptoms	+	+	0
Number of psychological symptoms resulting in a physician visit	+	+	0
Talked to doctor about emotional problems	+	+	0
Used specialty mental-health services	+	0	0

[a]Four or more unexplained symptoms and 3 or more on the Illness Worry Scale compared with nonsomatizers (less than 4 unexplained symptoms and less than 3 on the Illness Worry Scale).
[b]Four or more unexplained symptoms and less than 3 on the Illness Worry Scale compared with nonsomatizers.
[c]Less than four unexplained symptoms and 3 or more on the Illness Worry Scale compared with nonsomatizers.
[d]Table entries indicate positive relationship with the characteristic (+) and no relationship (0). Strong relationship indicated by double symbol (+ +).

considerable demands on the health care system, exceeded only by the demands made by functional somatizers who also held strong hypochondriacal beliefs. Hypochondriacal somatizers, however, made no more use of health services than nonsomatizers, perhaps because many suffered only from transient hypochondriacal worry (see Kellner, Chapter 8, this volume for a typology of hypochondriasis).

Because presenting somatizers make no connection between their psychiatric disorder and the somatic complaints they present to the doctor, it is likely that their psychiatric problems will remain unnoticed. Unrecognized psychiatric morbidity may increase subsequent health care utilization and result in costly investigations, interventions, and consultations with specialists (Goldberg and Bridges 1988; Katon et al. 1982; Smith et al. 1986). It is not known, however, whether presenting somatizers continue to report somatic complaints to the exclusion of psychiatric distress or, over time, come to acknowledge and report a psychological basis for their distress.

We compared the illness behavior of true, facultative, and initial somatizers with psychosocial presenters as defined above. If somatizers continued to focus on somatic distress over the follow-up year, we expected that they would exhibit greater utilization for physical health reasons and less utilization for psychological reasons than would psychosocial presenters. Alternatively, presenting somatization may simply reflect patients who are earlier in the natural history of a major depressive episode (Cadoret et al. 1980; Widmer and Cadoret 1978; Wilson et al. 1983). In this case, somatizers would be expected to report more psychological complaints over the ensuing year and to utilize health services more for psychological reasons. Our findings support the first interpretation: presenting somatization as an enduring mode of distress. Although there were no differences among groups in presentations for somatic symptoms, somatizers reported fewer, not more, new psychological symptoms ($F(3, 133) = 4.2$, $P = .007$), and fewer psychological symptoms that resulted in a physician visit ($F(3, 133) = 6.6$, $P < .003$) than did psychosocial presenters. Somatizers were also less likely than psychosocial presenters to have used specialty mental health services ($\chi^2(3) = 24.8$, $P < .001$), or to have talked to a doctor about emotional problems ($\chi^2(3) = 15.8$, $P = .001$). Thus, among patients with concurrent psychiatric problems, those who initially presented with exclusively somatic complaints continued to make fewer requests for psychiatric care over the ensuing year than did those who presented with psychiatric symptoms.

CONCLUSIONS

By deconstructing somatization into its components, as we have done in this chapter, we have learned that sociodemographic characteristics of one form do not necessarily correspond to those of another; that psychological processes of attention, recognition and attribution are present in varying degrees in different forms; and that the exaggerated illness behavior thought to be typical of somatizers is most characteristic of those patients meeting criteria for both functional and hypochondriacal somatization.

We have found, for example, that it is difficult to offer a single demographic profile of the typical somatizer. Functional somatizers were more likely to be female, unmarried, older, of lower socioeconomic positions, and urban residents. Hypochondriacal somatizers, while also likely to be of lower socioeconomic positions, were no more likely to be women than men, unmarried than married, or older than younger. They, as opposed to functional somatizers, were less likely to be working and more likely to be immigrants to North America. Presenting somatizers were indistinguishable from patients with psychiatric disorder who presented psychosocial complaints in terms of age, income, education, marital status, and immigration status, but were less likely to be female. The social dynamics and cognitive processes that explain why gender, marital status, and social position are related in different ways to different forms of somatization remain to be specified.

Deconstructing somatization alerts us to the psychological factors unique to specific forms of somatization and to the potential clinical consequences of mistaking one form for another. Hypochondriacal somatizers were strongly influenced by negative affectivity, but functional or presenting somatizers were not. In addition to worry about illness, hypochondriacal somatizers had a particularly pessimistic, foreboding view of themselves and the world. Yet, while being conscious of the vulnerability of their bodies and preoccupied with illness, they made no unusual demands for health care. Contrary to other somatizers, those with hypochondriacal beliefs without a co-occurring history of functional symptoms may be less of an economic burden and less at risk for iatrogenic injury than is often thought. The opposite problem—that physicians may view the complaints of hypochondriacal somatizers as being unjustified and so ignore them—may also be uncommon. There is some evidence that physicians do not notice when patients with high levels of illness worry are presenting with exaggerated symptoms (Mabe et al. 1988). Illness worry in itself, then, appears to have fewer consequences for the health system, practitioner, and individual than previously expected. Hypochondriacal somatization may become a serious clinical problem only when it does not respond to repeated reassurances by physicians or is associated with persistent and disabling physical symptoms.

Symptom attribution processes best distinguish presenting somatizers from patients who psychologize psychiatric disorders. Presenting somatizers do not connect somatic and intrapsychic distress. This characteristic may reflect psychological defenses against acknowledging a frightening and stigmatizing psychiatric illness, or a heightened sensitivity to norms discouraging emotional expression. Alternatively, these patients may be suffering from a psychiatric disorder qualitatively different in some respects from that found in specialized mental health settings. Although they may meet diagnostic criteria for current major depression or anxiety disorder, many presenting somatizers do not report high levels of dysphoria on self-report measures. Because patients with these disorders may not find their way into psychiatric clinics, we should consider, as have others (e.g., Shepherd and Wilkinson 1988), whether psychiatric disorders presenting to primary care are distinct from disorders that have been identified, described, and objectified by observations of patients who have requested psychiatric care.

In many ways the most problematic form of somatization—and the one that contributes most to clinical stereotypes—involves patients with a history of multiple medically unexplained somatic symptoms who also hold the belief that they are vulnerable to illness. As we have shown, patients who display both functional and hypochondriacal somatization are most likely to continue to utilize health services at a high rate, continue to present symptoms that receive no diagnosis, and continue to be hospitalized. In addition to the economic burden they represent, their quest for explanations may result in social rejection. As Lennon et al. (1989) have noted, patients with unexplained symptoms may be motivated to "doctor shop" and use services in order to obtain social validation for distress that exists only at a subjective level. Ironically, the more these patients seek a definite diagnosis and the more they endure treatments that fail, the less convinced others become that the distress is real or that the patients truly want to get better.

Physicians who confuse forms of somatization may leave the patient with a distinctly unsatisfactory impression of the interaction. Simon (Chapter 3, this volume) and Lennon et al. (1989) have written of the feeling of being profoundly misunderstood that somatizing patients sometimes experience when offered a psychiatric explanation for their distress. By differentiating functional from presenting somatizers, we can begin to understand how such an interpretation could do a disservice to some patients. Presenting somatizers, by our definition, have a concurrent psychiatric disorder, whereas the majority of functional somatizers do not. Only a third of the functional somatizers in our study received a lifetime psychiatric diagnosis of mood or anxiety disorder. Thus, the assumption that somatizers have an underlying major psychiatric disorder that accounts for their physical distress is more often wrong than right. Even when depression exists concurrently with somatic symptoms, as it does among presenting somatizers, the dysphoria may often be understood by patients as a consequence, not a cause, of their physical distress (Lennon et al. 1989). Goldberg and Bridges (1988) go further to suggest that somatization allows those who are unsympathetic to psychiatric illness (or who live in such a social context) to occupy the sick role when they are psychologically ill. Somatic symptoms may also provide a safe strategy for the weak and powerless to protest social inequities (Kleinman 1986). Thus, while somatization may represent hidden psychiatric morbidity, it may also be unrelated to psychiatric disorder or a defense against being forced to acknowledge unacceptable psychological or social conflicts.

In concluding, we should caution that the components of somatization we have identified in this chapter may reflect differing temporal characteristics of measurement. Functional somatization was defined as the lifetime history of unexplained somatic distress; presenting somatization reflects a current instance of somatized depression; hypochondriacal somatization combines state and trait, including individuals with either transient or persistent worry. In the extreme, functional somatization becomes DSM-III-R somatization disorder (American Psychiatric Association 1987). This condition is characterized by an extended history of multiple unexplained physical symptoms over multiple bodily systems. Features attributed to functional somatizers in cross-sectional studies may be closer to factors that perpetuate somatization than to those that cause it (Goldberg and Bridges 1988). In contrast to functional somatization, which may represent a lifetime-prevalence measure, presenting somatization can be seen as an incidence construct. Comparisons are then made between patients who somatize an acute depressive episode and those who psychologize their distress. Hypochondriacal somatization can be seen either as an enduring trait of body and illness preoccupation similar to Kellner's (see Chapter 8, this volume) "developmental hypochondriasis," or a transient state of illness worry similar to Kellner's "hypochondriacal reaction" and Barsky and colleagues' (1990) "transient hypochondriasis." Longitudinal studies are needed to distinguish the evolving components of the somatization process from the stable components of the somatization trait. We are currently engaged in such a study.

REFERENCES

American Psychiatric Association: Diagnostic and Statistical Manual of Medical Disorders, 3rd Edition, Revised. Washington, DC, American Psychiatric Association, 1987

Angel R, Thoits P: The impact of culture on the cognitive structure of illness. Cult Med Psychiatry 11:465–494, 1987

Barsky AJ, Klerman GL: Overview: hypochondriasis, bodily complaints, and somatic styles. Am J Psychiatry 140:273–283, 1983

Barsky AJ, Wyshak G: Hypochondriasis and related health attitudes. Psychosomatics 30:412–420, 1989

Barsky AJ, Wyshak G, Klerman G: Hypochondriasis—an evaluation of the DSM-III criteria in medical outpatients. Arch Gen Psychiatry 43:493–500, 1986

Barsky AJ, Geringer E, Wool CA: A cognitive-educational treatment for hypochondriasis. Gen Hosp Psychiatry 10:322–327, 1988a

Barsky AJ, Goodson JD, Lane RS, et al: The amplification of somatic symptoms. Psychosom Med 50:510–519, 1988b

Barsky AJ, Wyshak G, Klerman GL: Transient hypochondriasis. Arch Gen Psychiatry 47:746–752, 1990

Bart P: Social structure and vocabularies of discomfort: what happened to female hysteria? J Health Soc Behav 9:188–193, 1968

Beaber RJ, Rodney WM: Under diagnosis of hypochondriasis in family practice. Psychosomatics 25:39–45, 1984

Bishop GD: Gender, role, and illness behavior in a military population. Health Psychol 3:519–534, 1984

Blacker CVR, Clare AW: Depressive disorder in primary care. Br J Psychiatry 150:737–751, 1987

Bridges KW, Goldberg DP: Somatic presentation of DSM-III psychiatric disorders in primary care. J Psychosom Res 29:563–569, 1985

Cadoret RJ, Widmer RB, Troughton EP: Somatic complaints: harbinger of depression in primary care. J Affective Disord 2:61–70, 1980

Cannon WB: Bodily Changes in Pain, Hunger, Fear and Rage (1929). New York, Harper & Row, 1963

Costa PT Jr, McCrae RR: Hypochondriasis, neuroticism, and aging: when are somatic complaints unfounded? Am Psychol 40:19–28, 1985

Craig KD: Social modeling influences on pains, in The Psychology of Pain. Edited by Sternbach R. New York, Raven, 1978, pp 73–109

Crandell DL, Dohrenwend BP: Some relations among psychiatric symptoms, organic illness, and social class. Am J Psychiatry 123:1527–1537, 1967

Croyle RT, Uretsky MB: Effects of mood on self-appraisal of health status. Health Psychol 6:239–253, 1987

Eaton WW, Kessler LG (eds): Epidemiologic Field Methods in Psychiatry. Orlando, FL, Academic, 1985

Escobar JI: Cross-cultural aspects of the somatization trait. Hosp Community Psychiatry 38:174–180, 1987

Escobar JI, Burnam A, Karno M, et al: Somatization in the community. Arch Gen Psychiatry 44:713–718, 1987a

Escobar JI, Golding JM, Hough RL, et al: Somatization in the community: relationship to disability and use of services. Am J Public Health 77:837–840, 1987b

Escobar JI, Rubio-Stipec M, Canino G, et al: Somatic Symptom Index (SSI): a new and abridged somatization construct. J Nerv Ment Dis 177:140–146, 1989

Fava GA, Pilowsky I, Peirfedrici A, et al: Depressive symptoms and abnormal illness behavior in general hospital patients. Gen Hosp Psychiatry 4:171–178, 1982

Fenigstein A, Scheier MF, Buss AH: Public and private self-consciousness: assessment and theory. J Consult Clin Psychol 43:522–527, 1975

Goldberg DP, Bridges K: Somatic presentations of psychiatric illness in primary care setting. J Psychosom Res 32:137–144, 1988

Grings WW, Dawson ME: Emotions and Bodily Responses. New York, Academic, 1978

Hamilton M: Frequency of symptoms in melancholia (depressive illness). Br J Psychiatry 154:201–206, 1989

Hanback JW, Revelle W: Arousal and perceptual sensitivity in hypochondriasis. J Abnorm Psychol 87:523–530, 1978

Hansell S, Mechanic D: The socialization of introspection and illness behavior, in Illness Behavior: A Multidisciplinary Model. Edited by McHugh S, Vallis TM. New York, Plenum, 1986, pp 253–260

Helman CG: Psyche, soma and society: the social construction of psychosomatic disease. Cult Med Psychiatry 9:1–26, 1985

Joyce PR, Bushnell JA, Walshe JWB, et al: Abnormal illness behaviour and anxiety in acute non-organic abdominal pain. Br J Psychiatry 149:57–62, 1986

Katon W: The epidemiology of depression in medical care. Int J Psychiatry Med 17:93–112, 1987

Katon W, Kleinman A, Rosen G: Depression and somatization: a review. Am J Med 72:127–135, 241–247, 1982

Katon W, Ries RK, Kleinman A: The prevalence of somatization in primary care. Compr Psychiatry 25:208–215, 1984a

Katon W, Ries RK, Kleinman A: A prospective DSM-III study of 100 consecutive somatization patients. Compr Psychiatry 25:305–314, 1984b

Katon W, Vitaliano PP, Russo J, et al: Panic disorder: spectrum of severity and somatization. J Nerv Ment Dis 175:12–19, 1987

Kellner R: Functional somatic symptoms and hypochondriasis: a survey of empirical studies. Arch Gen Psychiatry 42:821–833, 1985

Kellner R: Psychological measurements in somatization and abnormal illness behavior. Adv Psychosom Med 17:101–118, 1987

Kellner R, Schneider-Braus K: Distress and attitudes in patients perceived as hypochondriacal by medical staff. Gen Hosp Psychiary 10:157–162, 1988

Kellner R, Abbott P, Pathak D, et al: Hypochondriacal beliefs and attitudes in family practice and psychiatric patients. Int J Psychiatry Med 13:127–139, 1983

Kenyon FE: Hypochondriacal states. Br J Psychiatry 129:1–14, 1976

Kirmayer LJ: Culture, affect and somatization. Transcultural Psychiatric Research Review 21:159–188, 1984

Kirmayer LJ: Somatization and the social construction of illness experience, in Illness Behavior: A Multidisciplinary Model. Edited by McHugh S, Vallis TM. New York, Plenum, 1986, pp 111–123

Kirmayer LJ: Languages of suffering and healing: alexithymia as a social and cultural process. Transcultural Psychiatric Research Review 24:119–136, 1987

Kirmayer LJ, Robbins JM: Three forms of somatization in primary care: prevalence, co-occurrence and sociodemographic characteristics. J Nerv Ment Dis (in press)

Kleinman A: Social Origins of Distress and Disease. New Haven, CT, Yale University Press, 1986

Lennon MC, Link BG, Marbach JJ, et al: The stigma of chronic facial pain and its impact on social relationships. Social Problems 36:117–134, 1989

Lipowski ZJ: Somatization: the concept and its clinical application. Am J Psychiatry 145:1358–1368, 1988

Mabe PA, Hobson DP, Jones LR, et al: Hypochondriacal traits in medical patients. Gen Hosp Psychiatry 10:236–244, 1988

Mandler G: Mind and Body: Psychology of Emotion and Stress. New York, WW Norton, 1984

Mathew RJ, Largen J, Claghorn JL: Biological symptoms of depression. Psychosom Med 41:439–443, 1979

McCrae RR, Costa PT Jr: Social desirability scales: more substance than style. J Consult Clin Psychol 51:882–888, 1983

Mechanic D: The influence of mothers on their children's health attitudes and behavior. Pediatrics 33:444–453, 1964

Merskey HA, Evans PR: Variations in pain complaint threshold in psychiatric and neurologic patients with pain. Pain 1:59–72, 1975

Miller LC, Murphy R, Buss AH: Consciousness of body: private and public. J Pers Soc Psychol 41:397–406, 1981

Pennebaker JW: The Psychology of Physical Symptoms. New York, Springer, 1982

Pennebaker JW, Lightner J: Competition of internal and external information in an exercise setting. J Pers Soc Psychol 39:165–174, 1980

Pennebaker JW, Skelton JA: Psychological parameters of physical symptoms. Personality and Social Psychology Bulletin 4:524–530, 1978

Pilowsky I: Dimensions of hypochondriasis. Br J Psychiatry 113:89–93, 1967

Pilowsky I, Spence ND: Patterns of illness behaviour in patients with intractable pain. J Psychosom Res 29:279–287, 1975

Pilowsky I, Spence ND: Manual for the Illness Behaviour Questionnaire (IBQ), Second Edition. Adelaide, Australia, University of Adelaide, 1983

Pilowsky I, Murrell GC, Gordon A: The development of a screening method for abnormal illness behaviour. J Psychosom Res 23:203–207, 1979

Pilowsky I, Bassett DL, Begg MW, et al: Childhood hospitalization and chronic intractable pain in adults: a controlled retrospective study. Int J Psychiatry Med 12:75–84, 1982

Pilowsky I, Smith QP, Katsikitis M: Illness behaviour and general practice utilization: a prospective study. J Psychosom Res 31:177–183, 1987

Radloff LS: The CES-D scale: a self-report depression scale for research in the general population. Applied Psychological Measurement 1:385–401, 1977

Robbins JM, Kirmayer LJ: Illness cognition, symptom reporting and somatization in primary care, in Illness Behavior: A Multidisciplinary Model. Edited by McHugh S, Vallis TM. New York, Plenum, 1986, pp 283–302

Robbins JM, Kirmayer LJ: Physical and psychological attributions of common somatic symptoms: development of the Symptom Interpretation Questionnaire. Working Papers in Social Behavior. Montreal, Department of Sociology, McGill University, No 90-1, 1990

Robbins JM, Kirmayer LJ, Kapusta MA: Illness worry and disability in fibromyalgia syndrome. Int J Psychiatry Med 20:49–63, 1990

Roberts RE, Vernon SW: The Center for Epidemiologic Studies Depression scale: its use in a community sample. Am J Psychiatry 140:41–46, 1983

Robins L, Helzer JE, Croughan J, et al: National Institute of Mental Health Diagnostic Interview Schedule: its history, characteristics, and validity. Arch Gen Psychiatry 38:381–389, 1981

Rodin J: Somatopsychics and attribution. Pers Soc Psychol Bull 4:531–540, 1978

Schuessler K, Hittle D, Cardascia J: Measuring responding desirably with attitude-opinion items. Social Psychology 42:224–235, 1978

Schulberg HC, Burns BJ: Mental disorders in primary care: epidemiologic, diagnostic, and treatment research directions. Gen Hosp Psychiatry 10:79–87, 1988

Schwab JJ, Bell RA, Warheit GJ, et al: Some epidemiologic aspects of psychosomatic medicine. Int J Psychiatry Med 9:147–159, 1978

Schwartz GE, Davidson RJ, Goleman DJ: Patterning of cognitive and somatic processes in the self-regulation of anxiety: effects of meditation versus exercise. Psychosom Med 40:321–328, 1978

Sheperd M, Wilkinson G: Primary care as the middle ground for psychiatric epidemiology. Psychol Med 18:263–267, 1988

Shields SA: Reports of bodily changes in anxiety, sadness, and anger. Motivation and Emotion 8:1–21, 1984

Smith G, Monson R, Ray D: Psychiatric consultation in somatization disorder: a randomized controlled study. N Engl J Med 314:1407–1413, 1986

Stoeckle JD, Barsky AJ: Attributions: uses of social science knowledge in the doctoring of primary care, in The Relevance of Social Science for Medicine. Edited by Eisenberg L, Kleinman A. Dordrecht, The Netherlands, D Reidel, 1980, pp 223–240

Swartz M, Blazer D, George L, et al: Somatization disorder in a community population. Am J Psychiatry 143:1403–1408, 1986a

Swartz M, Blazer D, Woodbury M, et al: Somatization disorder in a U.S. Southern community: use of a new procedure for analysis of medical classification. Psychol Med 16:595–609, 1986b

Swartz M, Hughes D, Blazer D, et al: Somatization disorder in the community: a study of diagnostic concordance among three diagnostic systems. J Nerv Ment Dis 175:26–33, 1987

Swartz M, Blazer D, George L, et al: Somatization disorder in a southern community. Psychiatric Annals 18:335–339, 1988

Swartz M, Landerman R, Blazer D, et al: Somatization symptoms in the community: a rural/urban comparison. Psychosomatics 30:44–53, 1989

Turkat I, Kuczmierczyk AR, Adams HE: An investigation of the aetiology of chronic headache—the role of headache models. Br J Psychiatry 145:665–666, 1984

Verbrugge L: Gender and health: an update on hypotheses and evidence. J Health Soc Behav 26:157–177, 1985

Watson D, Clark LA: Negative affectivity: the disposition to experience aversive emotional states. Psychol Bull 96:465–490, 1984

Watson D, Pennebaker JW: Health complaints, stress and distress: exploring the central role of negative affectivity. Psychol Rev 96:234–254, 1989

Wessely S, Powell R: Fatigue syndromes: a comparison of chronic "postviral" fatigue with neuromuscular and affective disorders. J Neurol Neurosurg Psychiatry 52:940–948, 1989

Whitehead WE, Busch CM, Heller BR, et al: Social learning influences on menstrual symptoms and illness behavior. Health Psychol 5:13–23, 1986

Widmer RB, Cadoret RJ: Depression in primary care: changes in pattern of patient visits and complaints during a developing depression. J Fam Pract 7:293–302, 1978

Wilkinson SR: The Child's World of Illness. Cambridge, UK, Cambridge University Press, 1988

Wilson D, Widmer R, Cadoret R, et al: Somatic symptoms: a major feature of depression in a family practice. J Affective Disord 5:199–207, 1983

Ziesat HA: Correlates of the tourniquet ischemia pain ratio. Percept Mot Skills 47:147–150, 1978

Zonderman AB, Heft MW, Costa PT Jr: Does the Illness Behavior Questionnaire measure abnormal illness behavior? Health Psychol 4:425–436, 1985

Chapter 7

Somatization in Consultation-Liaison Psychiatry

Charles V. Ford, M.D., Pamela E. Parker, M.D.

The concept of somatization is an area of major concern to the consultation-liaison psychiatrist. Physicians who work in this medical subspecialty are confronted daily with diagnostic problems that require them to evaluate various multidetermined symptom complexes at the interface of medical-biological and psychological-social factors.

In order to understand the current direction of clinical interest and research in this area, a brief history of consultation-liaison psychiatry and of the concepts of somatization should prove useful. Recent excellent, more detailed reviews of this information are available (Greenhill 1977; Levy 1989; Lipowski 1986).[1]

Consultation-liaison psychiatry had its origins in the work of George Henry (1929), who described his experiences with psychiatric consultations on over 300 patients. He recommended that all general hospitals should have a psychiatric consultant on the staff. Later, the Rockefeller Foundation, under the leadership of Alan Gregg, provided generous grants to support psychiatric training and patient care in general hospital settings; eight outstanding medical centers were chosen for this experimental venture (Summergrad and Hackett 1987). This financial support was instrumental in establishing several consultation-liaison programs that remain preeminent in the field today.

The work of Dunbar (1935), which suggested that some personality features were associated with certain diseases, was followed by the fascinating hypotheses of Alexander (1950), who investigated how specific psychological conflicts in association with personality and stress might cause or precipitate certain diseases (e.g., rheumatoid arthritis or peptic ulcer). Research by pioneers such as Mirsky (1958) seemed to confirm these speculations and helped to fan enthusiasm

---

[1]The following brief summary is indebted to these fine reviews.

for the therapeutic promise of "psychosomatic medicine." "Psycho-somatic" services were developed as components of departments of psychiatry, and these services subsumed consultation functions.

By the late 1960s psychosomatic medicine services had given way to organized consultation-liaison psychiatry services. Although many of the activities (e.g., consultation) remained similar, several changes in approach had occurred:

1. The promise of therapeutic gains for "psychosomatic" disease by psychotherapy or psychoanalysis had not been realized; thus, there was less emphasis on this topic.
2. The advent of effective psychotropic medications made it possible to make therapeutic interventions for a wide range of psychiatric syndromes (from delirium to depression).
3. Psychiatrists became fascinated by the psychological aspects of new technological interventions such as open-heart surgery.
4. The nonspecific effect of stress in exacerbating most diseases studied was recognized.
5. There was an increasing recognition that the psychological profiles of the so-called psychosomatic diseases were characterized primari-ly by aspects of illness behavior (Drossman et al. 1988; Ford et al. 1986). These aspects of illness behavior include how a person perceives a bodily sensation (e.g., the question of amplification [Barsky 1979]), how a person may communicate psychological distress (e.g., the phenomenon of alexithymia[2] [Sifneos 1973]), and those factors that influence the extent to which a person may utilize medical care (Mechanic 1972).

Previous thinking about psychosomatic diseases suggested that certain specific psychopathological conditions or conflicts produced physical disease and/or that physical diseases produced secondary

---

[2]Alexithymia is a concept that initially had some promise to explain psychosomatic illness. Sifneos (1973) proposed that persons who did not have the capacity to use words to describe (and therefore discharge) their emotions might have increased physiological activity associated with affective states. This increased activity, in turn, would lead to the production of disease. Lesser et al. (1979) suggested that alexithymia is a valid entity but not specific to persons with either psychosomatic disease or somatization. However, persons who are depressed or anxious, and who cannot describe their feelings as emotions, may focus upon one of the physiological concomitants of these disorders (e.g., tachycardia). The patient then presents to a physician with somatic symptoms instead of psychological complaints (Ford 1986).

psychological effects (e.g., depression). Work by Drossman et al. (1988) indicated that patients with irritable bowel syndrome who sought medical care differed significantly from those who did not seek medical care. For example, scores on Minnesota Multiphasic Personality Inventory (MMPI) scales for depression, hypochondriasis, and hysteria were significantly elevated for those who sought treatment. Similarly, Ford et al. (1986) reported that depression and anxiety were not correlated with the degree of dysfunction in rheumatoid arthritis and fibromyalgia but that those affects appeared to play a role in medical utilization.

Somatization can be regarded as one form of abnormal illness behavior (Pilowsky 1969). Somatization is multidetermined, being influenced by perception, the capacity to communicate distress, cultural attitudes, stigmatization, and reinforcers such as disability payments (Ford 1986; Katon 1982; Lipowski 1988).

The term *somatization* is now used to describe patients who seek medical help for bodily symptoms *misattributed* by them to organic disease. It is the most common way for psychiatric disorders to present (Lloyd 1986; Murphy 1989). Thus, the consultation-liaison psychiatrist will be frequently asked to evaluate patients whose symptoms do not have a satisfactory medical explanation.

CURRENT APPROACHES IN CONSULTATION-LIAISON PSYCHIATRY

During the past 10 to 20 years consultation-liaison psychiatry has focused on several areas:

1. A continuing interest in general hospital consultations, looking at who refers which patients for what problems. Techniques of consultation and the effectiveness of such interventions have also been investigated.
2. The development of "bridging" inpatient units that incorporate both medical and psychiatric treatment capabilities. These programs have been colloquially termed "med-psych units."
3. The establishment of outpatient consultation and treatment programs that attempt to serve patients who have combined medical and psychiatric problems and/or who display health care–seeking behavior in the absence of significant objective evidence of disease (i.e., somatization).
4. Liaison relationships with "high-tech" medical-surgical problems, particularly in the area of artificial life support mechanisms such as hemodialysis and implanted defibrillators or in areas such as organ transplantation, oncology, and AIDS.

The remainder of this chapter will primarily be concerned with the first three areas mentioned above.

General Hospital Psychiatric Consultations

Despite the high prevalence of psychiatric problems among general hospital inpatients, a relatively small proportion of these patients are referred for psychiatric consultation (Maguire et al. 1975). Depending on the type of hospital involved and the service (e.g., medicine or surgery), referral rates vary widely (Bustamente and Ford 1981). It is apparent that selective factors influence decisions to seek psychiatric consultation, and therefore it is probable that the distribution of psychiatric disorders observed by the psychiatric consultant is not representative of the general hospital population as a whole.

From our experience it would appear that those patients who are more often referred for psychiatric consultation are those who are problematic because of their behavior or who make physicians uncomfortable because of their overt displays of emotion (e.g., crying). Patients who are quietly depressed or apathetically delirious are less likely to attract attention.

Prevalence of Somatoform Disorders in Consultation-Liaison Practice

Those patients who are seen in psychiatric consultation are most frequently diagnosed as having organic or mood disorders. Relatively few are assigned a primary diagnosis of a somatoform disorder. However, one complicating factor in evaluating somatization in reported series of consultations has been the repeated changes in diagnostic terminology and criteria. To further complicate matters, various authors have grouped their diagnoses differently, thereby making it difficult to compare one series with another. The following experiences of general consultation services are representative of the psychiatric literature in this area.

At the Yale University–New Haven Hospital, Kligerman and McKegney (1971) reported a consultation rate of 2.9%. Of their consultation patients, 11.5% were diagnosed as having conversion reactions and 8.8% as having classical psychosomatic disease. (These percentages pertain to a time when the diagnostic criteria for conversion disorder were broader, but they still seem high compared with those in the reports discussed below.)

Bustamente and Ford (1981) noted that 2.0% of their consultations were diagnosed as having conversion disorder and 6.6% as having pain syndromes, and of all consultations only 13.2% (including the above) were considered to have a significant psychosomatic component. The consultation rate for the entire hospital during the period of investigation was approximately 2.8%.

Shevitz et al. (1976) reported that 5.6% of their consultations had a diagnosis of conversion disorder and 2.1%, a diagnosis of psychophysiological reactions. The consultation rate during the period of study was approximately 3%.

Taylor and Doody (1979) reported a consultation rate of 1.26% of all admissions at a Canadian hospital. Of these consultation patients, 8.4% were diagnosed as having conversion-type neurosis and 3% as having psychophysiological disorders.

Zuo and colleagues (1985) described a consultation service at a hospital in Hunan, China. Their consultation rate was 0.74% of admissions. They found that 5.3% of their consultation patients were diagnosed as having "hysteria" and another 5.3% as having "psychalgia" (presumably equivalent to somatoform pain disorder). Neurasthenia (mostly major depression by DSM-III criteria) accounted for another 12% of their consultations.

Fava and Pavan (1980) reported that at the University of Padua Medical Center in Italy, 1.2% of their consultation patients were diagnosed as having hysteria and another 6.0% as having psychophysiological reactions. No consultation rate was provided.

Snyder and Strain (1989) reviewed a series of 1,801 consultations at Mount Sinai Hospital in New York. They found that only 2.6% of the final diagnoses met the criteria for DSM-III somatoform disorders. Of these, conversion disorder was the most common. Those patients having somatoform disorders were more likely than other patients in the series to be female, Hispanic, and to have DSM-III Axis II comorbidity (48.5% vs. 20.7%). A physical disease (Axis III diagnosis) was present in 93% of these patients. These authors noted the low incidence of somatoform disorders as compared with other series, and the high comorbidity with physical disease. They suggested that these findings might reflect the very rigid requirements for admission to a hospital in the New York area.

Some other reports describing the diagnostic breakdowns of their consultations have not listed somatoform disorders. Presumably these disorders occurred too infrequently to warrant mention (Craig 1982; Hengeveld et al. 1984; Malhotra and Malhotra 1984).

From the above it would appear that conversion disorder is the most commonly diagnosed specific somatoform disorder by consultation-liaison psychiatrists working in general hospitals. Folks et al. (1984) looked at conversion disorder in a general hospital (Vanderbilt Medical Center). From their series of 1,000 consecutive consultations, 50 patients (5%) were diagnosed as having conversion disorder. An additional 12 patients, for whom psychiatric consultation had not been requested, were identified (by the hospital's computerized discharge diagnosis records) as having been discharged from the hospital with the diagnosis of conversion disorder during the same time period. When compared to other consultation patients, conversion patients, at a highly statistically significant level, were from a lower socioeconomic status and were more apt to come from a rural (versus an urban) background. No significant differences in sex, age, race, or education were found. Of importance, among the consultations on conversion patients, 60% of the patients had a concurrent psychiatric diagnosis (34% of the series met the DSM-III criteria for somatization disorder) and 20% had a concurrent neurological disorder. From these data and reports of other series of conversion patients, Ford and Folks (1985) opined that conversion should be considered a symptom rather than a diagnosis. They reasoned that conversion phenomenology occurs in a wide spectrum of psychiatric disorders from schizophrenia to depression, and is nonspecifically associated with neurological disease. Treatment is similarly nonspecific, and most conversion symptoms are transient and resolve spontaneously.

Although the various series of consultations reported above did not specifically mention somatization disorder, there is some evidence that it is fairly prevalent among hospitalized patients, but unrecognized and/or not diagnosed. De Gruy et al. (1987) found that of a sample of 213 hospitalized medical-surgical patients, 9% met the criteria for somatization disorder. Seventy-four percent of these somatization disorder patients had no objective findings by the time of their discharge to explain their symptoms. Further, none of the somatization disorder patients had been diagnosed as such by time of discharge. However, the finding that may be even more striking is the fact that 21% of the control group also did not have any physical evidence of disease. This finding suggests that there may be a significant reservoir of other types of somatization in hospitalized patients. One might speculate that this group includes such conditions as somatized depression or anxiety (Katon 1982, 1984).

Katon et al. (1984) investigated somatization in 261 consultation patients using a broad-based definition. These authors found that 100 of the consultation patients (38.3%) demonstrated somatization that was highly associated with major depression. Of their total sample of 261 patients, 12 (4.6%) had conversion disorder, 11 (4.2%) had psychogenic pain, and 4 (1.5%) had a factitious disorder.

Summary

From the foregoing review of somatization of general hospital consultation psychiatry, several conclusions emerge:

1. A significant portion of general hospital patients with psychiatric morbidity are not referred for psychiatric consultation.
2. This psychiatric morbidity may be disguised (or "masked") by somatization.
3. Those patients who are seen by consultation psychiatrists are not frequently diagnosed as having a somatoform disorder. Yet, many of the patients display some aspect of somatization in a nonspecific manner.
4. When a somatoform disorder (e.g., conversion) is diagnosed, it is likely to be associated with either psychiatric or physical comorbidity.

TREATMENT PROGRAMS FOR SOMATOFORM DISORDERS

Consultation-Liaison Outpatient Services

Several consultation-liaison psychiatric services have established outpatient clinics (Wolcott et al. 1984). These programs are highly varied one from another, but, in general, they have attempted to provide diagnostic and therapeutic psychiatric services to patients who have identified themselves as being physically sick. For example, the consultation-liaison psychiatrist might treat depression (comorbidity) in a patient with diabetes or anxiety in a patient with coronary artery disease. A significant portion of patients seen in consultation-liaison clinics are those who, despite their perception of organic illness, have relatively little in the way of objective findings to explain their physical symptoms. These patients, so-called "somatizers," fit the diagnostic criteria of the somatoform disorders to varying degrees.

As of their 1984 review, Wolcott et al. indicated that only eight reports had been published describing consultation-liaison clinics. Each of these clinics differed in many respects, and it is therefore difficult to characterize them. Most used various euphemisms for the clinic's name, apparently to make referral more acceptable to a nonpsychologically minded patient population.

Hunter and Lyon (1951) reported on the establishment of "Clinic H." for treatment of hypochondriacal patients. The clinic was established in an area adjacent to the main medical clinic, and the professional staff consisted of residents and faculty of the Division of

Psychosomatic Medicine (Psychiatry). Patients were seen supportively for relatively brief periods of time: 20 to 30 minutes at intervals from 1 week to 3 months. The treatment principles that they espoused included acceptance of the patient's complaints, willingness to examine the patient, polite interest, and the offer of a return appointment. Similar principles have more recently been proposed by other authors (Kutcher and Ford 1985; Smith et al. 1986) for patients who are treated in a primary care setting. Other more specific treatment approaches have been proposed for somatizing patients, and these are discussed elsewhere in this book (see Simon, Chapter 3; Kellner, Chapter 8; Kirmayer and Robbins, Chapter 10, this volume).

No specific follow-up data were provided for patients referred to Clinic H., but there was the impression that the approach was well accepted by both patients and physicians. A subsequent report on this clinic, 49 years after it was established (Ritvo and Thompson 1986), indicated that Clinic H. continued to be viable and a cost-effective mechanism for providing care for somatizing patients. These authors indicated that for the preceding 3 years only 2% to 5% of the Clinic H. patients required hospitalization as compared with 10% to 15% of the patients who attended the primary care medical clinic.

Lipsitt (1964) described the "Integration Clinic" of Boston's Beth Israel Hospital for the evaluation of dependent, depressed, multiple and vaguely symptomatic patients. Patients were seen for relatively few visits and usually referred back to their original clinic. Kaplan (1981) described a liaison clinic at Boston City Hospital. Of note, only 36 of the 83 patients who largely had somatization-type problems completed the evaluation process.

Rowan and colleagues (1984) established a liaison clinic at Mount Sinai Medical Center in New York. This clinic proposed to assess and treat patients with psychological problems related to physical complaints, including somatoform disorders. Treatment was multidisciplinary in nature and emphasized liaison with the referring clinic. Of interest, of the first 96 patients, only two had a DSM-III somatoform disorder diagnosis. The vast majority of patients fit into either a depressive or an anxiety spectrum syndrome.

One treatment program that may be associated with a consultation-liaison clinic is that of group therapy. Ford (1984) has suggested that some somatizing patients may be using medical care as an auxiliary social support system. Thus, if social support–oriented group therapy is provided, the need to repetitively present to medical-surgical clinics and emergency rooms may be obviated. Groups for these patients have been called in the literature such things as "treating the untreatables" (Mally and Ogston 1964). What is implied is that these patients are different from "psychiatric" patients and require different techniques. Somatizing patients may be described as "emotionally illiterate" (Mally and Ogston 1964) or "alexithymic" (Lesser et al. 1979; Sifneos 1973). They require a supportive rather than insight-oriented approach, and they usually do not respond well to emotional confrontations (Ford and Long 1977). However, these patients do demonstrate a significant reduction of medical utilization when engaged in treatment groups (Ford 1984).

In summary, it is difficult for somatizing patients to conceptualize their physical complaints in psychological terms. They are resistant to referrals to psychiatrically oriented clinics and may have difficulty participating in traditional psychotherapy. Thus, the strategies of placing consultation-liaison clinics in medical-surgical areas (vs. identified psychiatric space), utilizing relatively short interview sessions, and spacing time between visits are better accepted by patients and indeed may be more cost effective.

For those patients who will accept a referral to group therapy (and many will not), this particular treatment modality is very cost effective in reducing overall medical utilization.

Medical-Psychiatric Inpatient Services

The establishment of inpatient services ("med-psych" units) that attempt to respond to combined medical-psychiatric problems has to a large extent come from consultation-liaison psychiatry. Fogel and Goldberg (1983) suggested that certain groups of patients would be better served by having a consultation-liaison psychiatrist as the primary physician. These groups of patients included those with physical disease and psychiatric comorbidity, those with neurological disease and behavioral disturbances, mildly demented patients, patients with compliance problems, and patients who somatize. These somatizing patients may have genuine concurrent physical disease for which the symptoms are amplified, or may suffer from persistent medically unexplained symptoms.

Despite the appeal of Fogel and Goldberg's suggestions, with one exception (see below), medical-psychiatric units have not focused on somatization. The medical-psychiatric unit at St. Mary's Hospital, San Francisco, described by Hoffman (1984), cared for relatively few patients (6.5%) who were referred with a diagnosis of a somatoform disorder. Of these 14 patients, five had a referral diagnosis of conversion disorder, three were considered to be hypochondriacal, and two were labeled as having factitious disease or as malingering. Of interest, after a complete evaluation the discharge diagnoses changed in the direction of organic disease (Hoffman 1982). Three of the patients initially diagnosed with conversion were found to have a neurologic disease and one had factitious disease. Of those patients with psychogenic pain, two were found to have neurological disease, one was schizophrenic, and one had a diagnosis of analgesic dependence. A similar distribution of somatoform diagnoses was reported by Goodman (1985) at Mount Sinai Hospital. Of 266 admissions, six patients (2.1%) were diagnosed as having a factitious disorder and four patients (1.4%) as having a somatoform disorder.

The organization of the medical-psychiatric unit at Duke University Hospital may better facilitate the entry of somatizing patients into psychiatric care (Stoudemire et al. 1983). The Combined Medical Specialties Unit is a joint medical-psychiatric ward where every patient is admitted under the care of a faculty member of the Department of Medicine. At the time of admission each patient is also evaluated by a psychiatrist who specializes in the psychological aspects of medical illness. The treatment plan is developed jointly by the internist, psychiatrist, and nursing staff. If the psychiatric component of the patient's illness becomes the primary treatment focus, then the psychiatrist may become the attending physician. However, the internist remains involved to ensure that the patient does not feel abandoned.

In follow-up of the experiences with the Combined Medical Specialties Unit at Duke University Hospital, Stoudemire et al. (1985) reported their experience with over 200 patients admitted to the unit. After intensive psychiatric evaluation, over half received a depression-related diagnosis. Relatively few of these patients were initially diagnosed with a presumptive diagnosis of depression, but instead had presented to their internist with somatic complaints. The authors were less impressed with the alexithymic features of this group of patients than they were with characteristics described as rigid defense mechanisms or severe limitations in cultural, psychological, and educational development. The authors made the diagnosis of a somatoform disorder in only 5.5% of their patients. They suggested that a significant percentage of medical patients presumptively labeled "psychosomatic," "hysterical," "hypochondriacal," or "somatizing" actually suffer from underlying major mood disorders that require specific treatment.

Fogel et al. (1985) have compared the medical-psychiatric units at Duke and Brown Universities. The medical-psychiatric unit at Rhode Island Hospital (Brown University) is administratively and clinically different from that at Duke University in that it is organized under the auspices of psychiatry. This difference has been regarded as clinically advantageous because of a greater capacity for controlling agitated, psychotic, and suicidal behavior. The unit also offered more predictable payment for psychotherapy. Similar to the Duke University unit, the typical patient suffered from depression with prominent somatic symptoms. However, this type of unit organization (more psychiatrically oriented) may be less acceptable to some doctors and some patients. Referrals from the medical service at Duke University accounted for 50% of the admissions as opposed to only 20% of the admissions at Rhode Island Hospital. Patients who are fearful of stigma or who defend against the acceptance of a mental disorder may find a medically oriented unit less threatening.

In summary, clinical experience with combined medical-psychiatric units is still fairly exploratory. Initial experiences indicate that relatively few patients cared for by these units fit the usual criteria for somatoform disorders. Many of the patients have underlying depression that presents itself in the idiom of somatic symptoms. There is a suggestion that these patients find a medically oriented (vs. identified "psychiatric") treatment approach more acceptable.

CONCLUSIONS

The consultation-liaison psychiatrist, irrespective of the setting in which he or she works, will see a significant number of somatizing patients. Relatively few of these patients will strictly meet DSM-III-R criteria for somatoform disorders. Rather, they are typically depressed and/or anxious and present their distress to their physicians in a somatic idiom. On the whole they are resistant to being labeled as "psychiatric." Thus, effective therapeutic interventions require treating them in a medically oriented setting and employing different techniques from those used with more psychologically minded patients.

REFERENCES

Alexander F: Psychosomatic Medicine. New York, WW Norton, 1950

Barsky AJ: Patients who amplify bodily sensations. Ann Intern Med 91:63–70, 1979

Bustamente JP, Ford CV: Characteristics of general hospital patients referred for psychiatric consultation. J Clin Psychiatry 42:338–341, 1981

Craig TJ: An epidemiologic study of a psychiatric liaison service. Gen Hosp Psychiatry 4:131–137, 1982

De Gruy F, Crider J, Hashini DK, et al: Somatization disorder in a university hospital. J Fam Pract 25:579–584, 1987

Drossman DA, McKee DC, Sandler KS, et al: Psychosocial factors in the irritable bowel syndrome: a multivariate study of patients and non-patients with irritable bowel syndrome. Gastroenterology 95:701–708, 1988

Dunbar FH: Physical and mental relationships in illness. Am J Psychiatry 91:541–562, 1935

Fava GA, Pavan L: Consultation psychiatry in an Italian general hospital. Gen Hosp Psychiatry 2:35–40, 1980

Fogel BS, Goldberg RJ: Beyond liaison: a future role for psychiatry in medicine. Int J Psychiatry Med 13:185–192, 1983

Fogel BS, Stoudemire A, Houpt JL: Contrasting models for combined medical and psychiatric inpatient treatment. Am J Psychiatry 142:1085–1089, 1985

Folks DG, Ford CV, Regan W: Conversion symptoms in a general hospital. Psychosomatics 25:285–295, 1984

Ford CV: Somatizing disorders, in Helping Patients and Their Families Cope With Medical Problems. Edited by Roback HB. San Francisco, CA, Jossey-Bass, 1984, pp 39–59

Ford CV: The somatizing disorders. Psychosomatics 27:327–337, 1986

Ford CV, Folks DG: Conversion disorders: an overview. Psychosomatics 26:371–383, 1985

Ford CV, Long KD: Group psychotherapy of somatizing patients. Psychother Psychosom 28:294–304, 1977

Ford CV, Callahan LF, Brooks RH, et al: Psychological test results are not correlated with objective measure of function in rheumatoid arthritis, in Proceedings of the 15th European Conference on Psychosomatics Research. Edited by Lacey JH, Sturgeon DA. London, John Libbey, 1986, pp 303–306

Goodman B: Combined psychiatric-medical inpatient units: the Mount Sinai model. Psychosomatics 26:179–189, 1985

Greenhill MH: The development of liaison programs, in Psychiatric Medicine. Edited by Usdin G. New York, Brunner-Mazel, 1977, pp 115–191

Hengeveld MW, Rooymans HGM, Vecht-van der Bergh R: Psychiatric consultations in a Dutch university hospital: a report on 1,814 referrals, compared with a literature review. Gen Hosp Psychiatry 6:271–279, 1984

Henry GW: Some modern aspects of psychiatry in general hospital practice. Am J Psychiatry 86:481–499, 1929

Hoffman RS: Diagnostic errors in the evaluation of behavioral disorders. JAMA 248:964–967, 1982

Hoffman RS: Operation of a medical-psychiatric unit in a general hospital setting. Gen Hosp Psychiatry 6:93–99, 1984

Hunter H, Lyon J: Clinic H: haven for hypochondriacs. American Practitioner 2:67–69, 1951

Kaplan KH: Development of a psychiatric liaison clinic. Psychosomatics 22:502–512, 1981

Katon W: Depression: somatic symptoms and medical disorders in primary care. Compr Psychiatry 23:274–287, 1982

Katon W: Panic disorder and somatization: review of 55 cases. Am J Med 77:101–106, 1984

Katon W, Ries RK, Kleinman A: Part II: a prospective DSM-III study of 100 consecutive somatization patients. Compr Psychiatry 25:305–314, 1984

Kligerman MJ, McKegney FP: Patterns of psychiatric consultation in two general hospitals. Int J Psychiatry Med 2:126–132, 1971

Kutcher M, Ford CV: Diagnosis and management of the hypochondriacal patient. Compr Ther 11:54–58, 1985

Lesser I, Ford CV, Friedmann CT: Alexithymia in somatizing patients. Gen Hosp Psychiatry 1:256–261, 1979

Levy NB: Psychosomatic medicine and consultation-liaison psychiatry: past, present, and future. Hosp Community Psychiatry 40:1049–1056, 1989

Lipowski ZJ: Consultation-liaison psychiatry: the first half century. Gen Hosp Psychiatry 8:305–315, 1986

Lipowski ZJ: Somatization: the concept and its clinical application. Am J Psychiatry 145:1358–1368, 1988

Lipsitt DR: Integration clinic: an approach to the teaching and practice of medical psychology in an outpatient setting, in Psychiatry and Medical Practice in a General Hospital. Edited by Zinberg NE. New York, International Universities Press, 1964, pp 231–249

Lloyd GG: Psychiatric syndromes with a somatic presentation. J Psychosom Res 30:113–120, 1986

Maguire GP, Julier DL, Hawton KE, et al: Psychiatric morbidity and referral on two general medical wards. Br Med J 1:268–270, 1975

Malhotra S, Malhotra A: Liaison psychiatry in an Indian general hospital. Gen Hosp Psychiatry 6:266–270, 1984

Mally MA, Ogston WD: Treatment of the "untreatables." Int J Group Psychother 14:369–374, 1964

Mechanic D: Social psychologic factors affecting the presentation of bodily complaints. N Engl J Med 286:1133–1139, 1972

Mirsky IA: Physiologic, psychologic, and social determinants in the etiology of duodenal ulcer. American Journal of Digestive Diseases 3:285–313, 1958

Murphy M: Somatization: embodying the problem. Br J Med 298:1331–1332, 1989

Pilowsky I: Abnormal illness behavior. Br J Med Psychol 43:347–351, 1969

Ritvo JH, Thompson TL: A 49-year-old clinic for chronically ill somatizers. Hosp Community Psychiatry 37:631–633, 1986

Rowan GE, Strain JJ, Gise LH: The liaison clinic: a model for liaison psychiatry funding, training and research. Gen Hosp Psychiatry 6:109–115, 1984

Shevitz SA, Silberfarb PM, Lipowski ZJ: Psychiatric consultations in a general hospital: a report on 1,000 referrals. Diseases of the Nervous System 37:295–300, 1976

Sifneos PE: The prevalence of "alexithymic" characteristics in psychosomatic patients. Psychother Psychosom 22:255–262, 1973

Smith GR, Monson RA, Ray DC: Psychiatric consultation in somatization disorders: a randomized controlled study. N Engl J Med 314:1407–1413, 1986

Snyder S, Strain JJ: Somatoform disorders in the general hospital inpatient setting. Gen Hosp Psychiatry 11:288–293, 1989

Stoudemire A, Brown TJ, McLeod M, et al: The combined medical specialties unit: an innovative approach to patient care. NC Med J 44:365–367, 1983

Stoudemire A, Kahn M, Brown JT, et al: Masked depression in a combined medical-psychiatric unit. Psychosomatics 26:221–228, 1985

Summergrad P, Hackett TP: Alan Gregg and the rise of general hospital psychiatry. Gen Hosp Psychiatry 9:439–445, 1987

Taylor G, Doody K: Psychiatric consultations in a Canadian general hospital. Can J Psychiatry 24:717–723, 1979

Wolcott DL, Fawzy FI, Pasnau RO: Consultation-liaison outpatient clinics. Gen Hosp Psychiatry 6:153–161, 1984

Zuo C, Yang L, Chu CC: Patterns of psychiatric consultation in a Chinese general hospital. Am J Psychiatry 142:1092–1094, 1985

Chapter 8

Treatment Approaches to Somatizing and Hypochondriacal Patients

Robert Kellner, M.D., Ph.D., F.R.C.Psych.

I n this chapter I address the treatment of somatization and hypochondriasis using the classification described by Kirmayer and Robbins in Chapter 1 of this volume. This classification identifies three broad forms of somatization: somatic clinical presentations of psychiatric disorders; functional somatic symptoms or medically unexplained distress; and hypochondriasis, illness worry, or somatic preoccupation. This classification is new, and the research on the treatment of somatization is sparse. There has, however, been some progress in the knowledge of the nature of somatization and hypochondriasis during the last two decades, and it has outstripped our knowledge about treatment. Most of what we know of the treatment of somatization is derived from the treatment of specific functional somatic syndromes, some of which are described by Kirmayer and Robbins in Chapter 5 of this volume.

For the purpose of discussing treatment approaches, it is useful to further subdivide medically unexplained distress into isolated idiopathic symptoms, which may be transient or persistent, specific functional syndromes (e.g., irritable bowel, fibromyalgia, chronic fatigue) and high levels of generalized functional symptomatology (as in somatization disorder). Similarly, hypochondriasis may occur as a transient reaction, a persistent neurotic problem, or a chronic developmental pattern resembling a personality disorder. These different forms may require different modes and durations of treatment.

The recommendations about the treatment of somatization and hypochondriasis are tentative. They will change when new research becomes available, as will the recommendations about the appropriate treatment strategies for the three forms of somatization outlined in Chapter 1. In turn, the forms themselves are likely to be redefined.

Some general principles apply to the treatment of somatizing patients. In many cases the therapist will need to stay in touch and cooperate with the primary physician. The patient may need to be persuaded that psychological or psychiatric treatments are pertinent to patients with bodily ailments, and the therapist needs to accept the patient as someone who suffers rather than as a person whose symptoms satisfy unmet needs. Specific techniques for the treatment of various functional somatic symptoms and syndromes are described in the sections that follow.

SOMATIC PRESENTATION OF MOOD DISORDERS AND ANXIETY DISORDERS

The coexistence of somatic symptoms with mood disorders and anxiety disorders has been established in numerous studies (Kellner 1990), and treatment of this category is the most firmly established of any form of somatization. Somatic symptoms are more common in anxious and depressed patients than in nonanxious and non-depressed control subjects, and there is also strong evidence that the somatic symptoms decrease in most patients when the primary disorder wanes or is successfully treated. The somatic presentation of mood disorders and anxiety disorders may have prognostic implications. For example, the patient may pursue physical diagnosis and treatment, but the underlying mood disorder or anxiety disorder may be masked and remain inadequately treated. Controlled studies of drug treatment of mood disorders and anxiety disorders suggest that the appropriate treatment is effective regardless of whether the predominant presentation is emotional or somatic (Lipowski 1990).

FUNCTIONAL SOMATIC SYMPTOMS AND SYNDROMES

Isolated or Sporadic Functional or Idiopathic Symptoms

A substantial proportion of patients seek medical help for somatic symptoms for which no organic cause can be found (Kellner 1965; Mayou 1976). Although estimates have varied widely (Kellner 1986), the usual estimates on the proportion of these patients are in the range of 20% to 30%, depending on the type of practice, the thoroughness of the investigation, and the physician's diagnostic philosophy. Physicians differ in the extent to which they are willing to attribute a symptom or set of symptoms to a physical cause as opposed to concluding that it is functional. Where a psychosocial precipitant can be identified, many of these patients would be classified in DSM-III-R as having an adjustment disorder with physical complaints.

Considering the extent of the problem, the cost, and the implications for public health (Ford 1983; Kellner 1990), there are only a few studies on the prognosis of patients with sporadic functional somatic symptoms, and to my knowledge only one study has compared two different treatments in a controlled manner. Thomas (1978), in a family practice in Portsmouth, England, randomly assigned 200 patients in whom no definite diagnosis could be made to two different treatment procedures. Half were given a "symptomatic diagnosis and medication"; the others were told they had no evidence of disease and therefore required no treatment. From the description of complaints, it appears that these two groups of patients could have had either minor physical disorders or functional somatic symptoms, and probably both types of problems were included in each group. Seventy-one percent of the patients did not return for follow-up. But in those who did return, there was no significant difference between the two groups in the proportion who requested more treatment and in the proportion of who claimed they "felt better" (the latter representing more than 50% of those who returned for treatment). Because in the United Kingdom patients are registered with one family practitioner for all medical treatment, Thomas assumed that most of those who did not return did not feel in need of further treatment. In this study the diagnosis remained uncertain. Some of these patients may have had functional somatic symptoms that perhaps were associated with depression, anxiety, or adjustment disorder. Others may have had psychophysiological disorders or minor physical ailments such as viral infections, gastroduodenitis, and muscle sprains. This diagnostic uncertainty, however, applies to a large proportion of the symptoms encountered by primary care physicians that are judged to be functional, because, except for research purposes, extensive investigations—which are both costly and may involve risk—are not justified. Thus, the exact cause of short-lived symptoms often remains unknown. Thomas's study, however, shows that on follow-up the effect of medications was no different from the effect of reassurance and instructions among patients for whom "no definite diagnosis could be made." Recovery, judged by the method used in this study, was the same in both groups.

Although the duration of patients' symptoms in Thomas's study is not known, a tentative implication is that explanation and reassurance constitute adequate and appropriate treatment (Sapira 1972). In primary care the early management of functional somatic symptoms should combine frankness, explanation, and safety. The approach I advocate is slightly different from Thomas's. If the patient's symptoms are caused by depression or anxiety, these disorders may require specific treatment. If the patient does not have a conspicuous psychiatric disorder (Bridges and Goldberg 1985; Kessel 1960), the explanation should be as follows: "I can find no cause for the symptoms; it seems to me that it is a cramp [or another physiological explanation that is likely to be easily understood and does not frighten the patient], and I prefer not to treat it with drugs. If it does not get better, or if you have any other reason to be concerned, please come and see me again." It seems to me that without a thorough workup and reevaluation on follow-up, there is risk involved in telling a patient that there is no disease and that they therefore do not require treatment. Such a statement is sometimes wrong. There are numerous diseases that in the early stages can cause symptoms in the absence of abnormal physical signs or laboratory investigations (Kellner 1987). Consequently, premature and unqualified assurance could have a suggestive effect or induce a robust denial, and could make the patient desist from seeking treatment even after new symptoms of a dangerous disease appear. Nevertheless, Thomas's study shows that explanation and reassurance will be adequate in a large majority of patients with vague undiagnosable symptoms. In patients in whom symptoms persist or get worse, or in whom it becomes established that the symptoms are caused by one of the somatoform disorders, additional treatments (as described below) may become advisable.

Most psychiatrists do not carry out their own physical examination and laboratory investigations in patients who, in the course of psychiatric treatment, present new somatic symptoms. The approach that I recommend here for the primary care physician can also be modified and used by the treating psychiatrist after physical disease has been excluded.

Persistent Functional or Idiopathic Somatic Symptomatology

The most commonly encountered subgroup of somatoform disorders is the undifferentiated somatoform disorder of DSM-III-R (American Psychiatric Association 1987). (The relatively rare variant, somatization disorder, is discussed below in the section on chronic somatic complaints.) Whereas one of the DSM-III-R criteria for adjustment disorder with physical complaints is a duration of less than 6 months, an undifferentiated somatoform disorder typically lasts at least 6 months. Thus, the difference between undifferentiated somatoform disorder and the disorders described in the previous section is mainly one of duration.

A wide range of treatments have been suggested for somatization, and it is beyond the scope of the present chapter to enumerate them all (see Kellner 1986, pp. 12–14). In this century the efficacy of the treatment of somatizing patients has been underestimated for several reasons. Nonpsychiatric physicians found that many somatizing patients were resistant to conventional medical treatment, and psychiatrists formed their own opinions about the poor prognosis from chronic, unrepresentative patients who had been referred to them as a last resort after many years of failed medical treatment. Early studies of psychotherapy showed that somatizing patients respond less well to conventional insight psychotherapy than do patients with other emotional symptoms (Rosenberg 1954; Stone et al. 1965). Recent research, however, reveals a picture that is entirely different from the earlier one. There are now several controlled studies of patients presenting with functional bodily complaints who, two or three decades ago, would have been classified as "somatizers." Complaints such as muscle contraction headaches or nonulcer dyspepsia are today regarded as specific syndromes. In current diagnostic practice a few of these patients might be classified retrospectively as having undifferentiated somatoform disorders, while others might be classified in another category of DSM-III-R (e.g., psychological factors affecting physical condition).

PSYCHOTHERAPY AND BEHAVIOR THERAPY OF SPECIFIC FUNCTIONAL SYNDROMES

The work reviewed in this volume suggests that many of the complaints of somatizing patients could be regarded as incomplete manifestations of recognized functional somatic syndromes (see Kirmayer and Robbins, Chapter 5). Treatment of these patients is summarized below because these treatments are likely to be effective for somatizing patients in general. Not only is there evidence for the efficacy of psychotherapy in treating these somatizing patients, but evidence suggests that psychological treatments are more effective in patients with bodily complaints than in patients with psychic or overt emotional symptoms.

Headache

Numerous controlled studies of the treatment of headaches have been published. The pathology of migraine headaches differs substantially from that of other somatoform disorders. Muscle contraction headaches, however, are of importance because many somatizing patients have these headaches and the principles of the treatment of muscle contraction headaches are perhaps applicable to pain caused by excessive contraction of striated muscle in other parts of the body. Several reviewers have concluded that for muscle contraction or tension headaches, electromyographic biofeedback and muscle relaxation training were equally effective, and both treatments were superior to placebo treatment in short-term outcome ("Biofeedback and Tension Headache" 1980; Blanchard et al. 1988; Jessup et al. 1979; Nuechterlein and Holroyd 1980). In one study, stress-coping training was a more effective treatment than relaxation and biofeedback (Holroyd et al. 1977).

Irritable Bowel Syndrome and Other Gastrointestinal Syndromes

Treatment of the irritable bowel syndrome (IBS) is of importance for the understanding of the treatment of somatization in part because 1) the treatment of other functional gastrointestinal symptoms may be similar, 2) IBS is common, and 3) many of the gastrointestinal symptoms of somatizing patients may be partial or atypical manifestations of IBS (Cann and Read 1985).

Schonecke and Schüffel (1975), using a two-by-two design, evaluated the effects of brief psychotherapy and an experimental drug in treating IBS patients. No difference was found between psychotherapy and placebo. However, psychotherapy was remarkably brief: six sessions of 20 minutes each.

Whorwell et al. (1984) carried out a study of the use of hypnotherapy in treating IBS patients with severe refractory symptoms. Patients in the control group received a placebo and seven 30-minute sessions of supportive psychotherapy from a gastroenterologist. The sessions included "discussion of symptoms and an exploration of any possible contributory emotional problems and stressful life events" (p. 1232). The authors found that the psychotherapy group made small but statistically significant improvements in the symptoms that were evaluated, except for bowel habits, which remained unchanged. Hypnotherapy, which consisted of seven 30-minute sessions of decreasing frequency over a 3-month period, was solely directed at general relaxation and control of intestinal motility, and no attempt was made at hypnoanalysis. Following "general comments about improvement of health and wellbeing," the patient was asked to focus on "the control of intestinal smooth muscle" (p. 1232). The patient was given a simple account of intestinal smooth-muscle physiology. The patient was asked to use "reinforcement by visualization" (p. 1232) if he or she were able. In addition, "standard ego-strengthening suggestions" (p. 1232) were used at the end of each session. At the end of treatment, symptoms were either mild or absent in *all* 15 hypnotherapy patients.

Svedlund et al. (1983) carried out the largest and, thus far, best-designed study of psychotherapy in the treatment of IBS. The authors described their treatment as follows:

Psychotherapy, given in ten hour-long sessions spread over three months, aimed at modifying maladaptive behaviour and finding new solutions to problems. The focus was on means of coping with stress and emotional problems. Sometimes a more educative or teaching strategy about relations between stressful life events and abdominal symptoms was used. All psychotherapeutic measures were tailored to suit individuals and took the patients' tolerance of anxiety into account. (p. 589)

The mean number of sessions was 7.4, because several patients dropped out before the end of treatment. Both experimental and control groups improved, but the improvement in the psychotherapy group was significantly greater for abdominal pain and bowel dysfunction. This study was remarkable in that on follow-up, the difference in improvement between the experimental group and the control group increased, which is unusual in psychotherapy research. Often, differences found at the end of the treatment are no longer significant on follow-up.

It is of interest to compare the above three studies. Svedlund and his colleagues had the largest sample (over 50 in each group), and patients received the greatest number of psychotherapy sessions. In Whorwell et al.'s study the patients had seven 30-minute sessions of supportive psychotherapy with a small yet significant improvement. In Schonecke and Schüffel's study there was no improvement in the psychotherapy group compared with the placebo control group after six 20-minute sessions. Although it is inappropriate to assume that the skills and techniques of the therapists across these studies were identical, from the data thus far, one might argue that when the data are considered collectively, the authors of these three studies have established a dose-response curve. Perhaps the most impressive aspect of Svedlund et al.'s study is the finding that a few sessions of psychotherapy produced substantial changes and that the psychotherapy patients continued to improve on follow-up, whereas the patients treated with routine medical care deteriorated.

The findings of Whorwell et al. (1984) suggest that hypnotherapy might be a neglected method of treatment in patients with functional gastrointestinal disorder and perhaps in patients with functional disorders involving excessive smooth-muscle activity in other parts of the body.

Bates et al. (1988) examined the effects of a psychological treatment program for patients with dyspepsia without accompanying ulcers. The treatment was carried out in a group setting. The patients were asked to fill in a "pain diary" that included the situation in which the pain occurred, who was present at the time, the kind of physical activity, and other events. Throughout the program the patients were trained in applied relaxation (Ost 1988). Based on the information from the diary, the therapist, as well as group members, helped the patient to analyze the situation and to suggest alternative ways of behaving. Instructions for problem solving, assertiveness training, and cognitive restructuring were given to the patient to practice. At the end of the 3-month treatment, pain intensity and frequency were significantly less for treated patients than for control patients who used only the pain diary.

Sjödín et al. (1986) carried out a study of psychotherapy of patients with peptic ulcer. This study is pertinent to the treatment of somatization because the authors also examined the effects of psychotherapy on somatic symptoms that were unrelated to symptoms caused by ulcers. (The study was carried out by the same team that carried out the controlled study with IBS described above [Svedlund et al. 1983], and the design and treatment strategies were similar.) After the psychotherapy group had received an average of 7.6 sessions, there was a significantly greater improvement of somatic symptoms in general, and ulcer symptoms in particular, than in the medically treated group, and these differences in outcome were maintained on 15-month follow-up. Sjödín et al.'s study is another controlled study in which a small number of sessions of psychotherapy was associated with a significant and lasting improvement of somatic symptoms. Moreover, the symptoms were not limited to those of one psychosomatic disorder; instead, psychotherapy improved somatization in general.

Fibromyalgia-Fibromyositis

The fibromyalgia-fibromyositis syndrome consists of muscle pains, stiffness, tenderness at specific sites, and nonrestorative sleep. In the primary form of the disorder, no other disease is present to account for the symptoms. The more severe cases are associated with other stress disorders such as tension headaches, IBS, and chronic fatigue syndrome (CFS) (Yunus and Masi 1986).

In an early study, Draspa (1959) treated patients with muscular pain in whom no disease was found to account for the symptoms. Six sessions of psychological treatment combined with physiotherapy were compared with physiotherapy alone. The psychological treatment contained the following elements: reassuring the patients that the pain was only muscular and posed no danger; teaching the patients passive and active relaxation; and "giving insights into the causes of excessive muscular contraction" and so "promoting self-adjustment to change internal or external environmental situations." The combination of psychotherapy and physiotherapy was substantially more effective than physiotherapy alone in relieving idiopathic muscular pain.

Chronic Fatigue Syndrome

CFS is characterized by excessive fatigue, and viral infections often coincide with the onset of the syndrome. In many patients there is either evidence of persistent viral infection or immunological evidence of previous infections. A survey of the literature suggests that the etiology of the syndrome varies from one individual to the next, and in a majority of these individuals, physical and psychological symptoms interact (R. Kellner, manuscript in preparation). In an uncontrolled study, Wessely et al. (1989) treated patients having severe and chronic fatigue (average duration 4.5 years) in whom spontaneous recovery was judged to be unlikely. The treatment consisted of the establishment of a therapeutic relationship with the patient, treatment of a coexisting mood disorder, and a combined behavioral and cognitive approach that included guidance in gradually increasing physical activity and the assumption by the patient of new roles. A substantial proportion of the patients recovered or improved. While spontaneous recovery cannot be ruled out in an uncontrolled study, this explanation of the improvement seems unlikely in view of the chronicity and poor prognosis of the patients in this study.

DRUG TREATMENTS FOR FUNCTIONAL SOMATIC SYMPTOMS

Most patients with occasional functional somatic symptoms do not require drug treatment (Thomas 1978). Somatization that occurs in the course of either a mood disorder or an anxiety disorder is often relieved when the primary disorder is treated. For example, there is evidence from controlled double-blind drug trials that benzodiazepines, imipramine, phenelzine, and propranolol decrease somatic symptoms in anxious patients (Covi et al. 1974; Glass et al. 1987; Kahn et al. 1986; Sheehan et al. 1980; Tyrer 1976; Uhlenhuth et al. 1982). Similarly, in depressed patients, somatic symptoms decreased after treatment with tricyclic antidepressants (Covi et al. 1974) or monoamine oxidase inhibitors (Robinson et al. 1973). Psychotropic drugs have been found to be beneficial in various functional somatic disorders. For example, amitriptyline has been found to be effective in fibromyalgia (Goldenberg et al. 1986), while tricyclic antidepressants in general were found to be effective in several studies of headaches (Okasha et al. 1973). Desipramine was found to be effective in the treatment of IBS (Greenbaum et al. 1987).

The most appropriate indications and effective use of drug treatment for functional somatic symptoms have not been determined with certainty, and the drugs may have different effects in different disorders. In my experience there are large differences among individuals in therapeutic effects as well as in side effects. The mode of action is also uncertain. In some patients, drugs may exert their main effect by reducing anxiety and depression, thus secondarily reducing the severity of the bodily complaints. In these patients, when anxiety or depression decreases, so does the tendency for amplifying somatic distress (Barsky and Klerman 1983), as does the motive for selectively attending to bodily sensations. In others, for example, patients with myalgia or rheumatoid arthritis, the drugs may have an analgesic effect. In some patients the drugs may specifically modify the physiological abnormality. For example, in gastrointestinal syndromes such as IBS or one of its variants, small doses of desipramine are more effective than therapeutic doses of atropine, suggesting that a specific antimuscarinic effect may play a role (Greenbaum et al. 1987).

In patients in whom functional somatic symptoms persist, particularly if the patients are also anxious or depressed, and if psychotherapy has failed, drug treatment is indicated. Several different drugs may have to be tried before the most effective one is found. Drug treatment should not be continued if the drug does not clearly relieve symptoms.

SOMATIZATION DISORDER AND CHRONIC SOMATOFORM DISORDERS

Patients with *chronically* high levels of functional or idiopathic symptomatology may form a separate group. Little is known about the treatment of somatization disorder. Either the studies are retrospective (Coryell and Norten 1981; Guze and Perley 1963; Scallet et al. 1976) or there are limited, small control groups that are inadequate to judge the efficacy of treatment.

Yalom (1970) expressed the view that patients who somatize or "deal with . . . [problems] in a nonpsychological mode, are usually poor group referrals" (p. 175). He also cites results showing that somatizing patients are overrepresented among the dropouts from group therapy. These findings are similar to those of early studies of individual psychotherapy with somatizing patients that have been discussed above. Yalom apparently attempted to treat somatizing patients with group psychotherapy that did not specifically address the patients' somatic concerns. His results suggest that conventional nondirective, insight-oriented group psychotherapy may not be suitable for somatizing patients.

Valko (1976) reported a small, uncontrolled study of group therapy with six patients with Briquet's syndrome. The author reported that the patients improved fairly rapidly: their relationships with their families improved, the use of medication decreased substantially in most patients, and the number of visits to nonpsychiatric physicians decreased. Also, the patients reported that they had more self-confidence and that their mood had improved. Group therapy with these patients lasted for 4 months. Three of the patients relapsed but improved rapidly again when the group was restarted and treatment resumed. The patients improved quickly in several areas of their lives. (It should be kept in mind that this was a small, uncontrolled study.) This positive effect of psychotherapy is in contrast to the generally gloomy prognosis in patients with somatization disorder, with whom outcome studies indicate chronicity and poor response to treatment (Kellner 1988).

Recommendations for Treatment

In the absence of adequately controlled studies, any recommendations for treatment are, of course, tentative. The guidelines presented here are based on the experiences of therapists who have reported their findings, on the outcome of uncontrolled studies, and on the outcome of treatment of patients with similar disorders. These principles apply to all patients with chronic and distressing somatoform disorders. A brief summary of these strategies follows. (This treatment approach has been outlined in greater detail elsewhere [Kellner 1989b].)

The therapist must be prepared to accept the patient's description of pain and suffering. The patient may not believe that he or she is in need of psychiatric treatment, and the therapist will need to convey initially that the therapist's role is to help with the emotional consequences of having distressing bodily symptoms. Because the patient has persistent or recurring distressing bodily symptoms, including pain, the therapeutic approaches outlined in the previous sections should be tried. Coexisting disorders such as anxiety and depression often need to be treated with drug therapy. The therapist should try to persuade the patient to limit visits to one physician, thereby reducing the likelihood that multiple diagnoses and treatments will be offered (Ford 1983). Cooperation between the psychiatrist and the patient's primary physician substantially decreases the cost of medical investigations and probably also their risk (Smith et al. 1986). The primary physician should support the therapist's efforts, which may include weaning the patient from numerous inappropriate medications.

At present, except for isolated case histories (Patterson and Spees

1988), there are no published studies on family therapy in treating patients with somatoform disorders or in treating patients who chronically somatize. Family therapy may help the other family members to understand the disorder; it also may help them to tolerate the patient's behavior and to learn to respond more appropriately. Group psychotherapy deserves a trial when several patients with somatizing disorder or chronic somatic complaints present for treatment at the same time (Dwan and Nesbitt 1978; Ford and Long 1977; Mally and Ogston 1964).

There also are no adequate studies on drug treatment of chronically somatizing patients or of patients with somatization disorder. The main role of psychotropic drugs is the treatment of intercurrent or coexisting psychiatric disorders such as depression and anxiety. If antidepressants are prescribed, several attempts may be needed to find one that has the best therapeutic effects and the least unpleasant side effects, since some of these patients are exquisitely sensitive to new physical symptoms. Newer agents with less anticholinergic effects, such as trazodone or fluoxetine, may be helpful in this regard, but there are no adequately controlled studies with somatizing patients to date.

Patients with persistent functional somatic symptoms are at risk for the overprescription and overutilization of psychotropic drugs. The clinician must avoid the unnecessary use of drugs, particularly the long-term use of habit-forming drugs, and direct the patient toward other treatment modalities.

There are numerous studies that report the outcome of chronic somatizers—mainly patients with chronic pain—in units specializing in behavioral medicine or multidisciplinary pain treatment. There is no evidence at present that these units are superior to conventional treatments in chronic somatizers. Patients who do not respond to any treatment may be suffering from more complex or multiple disorders such as coexisting chronic mood disorders. The treatment of these patients is discussed below together with that of patients with chronic hypochondriasis.

HYPOCHONDRIASIS, ILLNESS WORRY, AND SOMATIC PREOCCUPATION

There are no adequate controlled studies of psychotherapy in the treatment of hypochondriasis. The studies that do exist either deal with similar conditions such as physical disease with hypochondriacal tendencies (Cooper et al. 1975) or have a design that is unsuitable for the evaluation of the effects of treatment (Kellner and Sheffield 1971).

Numerous and diverse treatments have been advocated in hypochondriasis, and there is substantial disagreement on the most suitable treatments (for review see Kellner 1986). Uncontrolled studies suggest that psychotherapy can change false beliefs about disease, attitudes, and behavior, and there is evidence that a substantial proportion of patients will improve or recover after psychotherapy (Kellner 1983; Pilowsky 1968).

Several attributes and behaviors constitute the hypochondriacal syndrome, including excessive worry about illness, unusual concern about pain, false beliefs of having a disease (i.e., disease conviction), excessive fear of disease (i.e., disease phobia), fear of death and thanatophobia, undue attendance to bodily sensations, amplification of bodily symptoms, excessive treatment experience, demands for medical investigations and care, and, yet, poor precautions about health (Barsky and Wyshak 1989; Kellner et al. 1987; Küchenhoff 1985). This syndrome in turn often coexists with other disorders such as depression and anxiety (Barsky et al. 1986; Kellner et al. 1989). Because of this comorbidity, more than one strategy of psychotherapy may have to be used.

The proposed psychotherapeutic approaches that are summarized here can be regarded only as guidelines. These approaches are based on uncontrolled outcome studies (Barsky et al. 1988a; House 1989; Kellner 1982) and on controlled studies of similar disorders including somatizing patients.

Psychotherapeutic Strategies in Hypochondriasis

Special efforts to negotiate with hypochondriacal patients may be required to engage them in therapy for their primary disorder. When hypochondriasis is secondary to another disorder such as melancholia or panic disorder, the primary disorder should be treated first. When the primary disorder is effectively treated, hypochondriacal fears and beliefs remit in a substantial proportion of patients (Kellner et al. 1986; Noyes et al. 1986), and no other treatment may be necessary.

Personalities, attitudes, and clinical features of hypochondriacal patients differ substantially, and therefore the same treatment is unlikely to be suitable for all. The treatment strategies and rationale have been described in detail elsewhere (Kellner 1989a).

In patients with recent and mild hypochondriacal reactions, examination and explanation of the nature of the symptoms are usually all that is required. Persistent, particularly long-standing hypochondriasis that has resisted all previous physicians' reassurances may pose a challenge to the therapist. Ladee (1966) described the outcome of a series of 23 cases treated with "uncovering" psychotherapy.

Most of the patients had analytically oriented psychotherapy, and a few had been treated with psychoanalysis. The group was selected for motivation, willingness to cooperate, and the absence of a long history of iatrogenic reinforcement. The results were "satisfactory to good" in only four cases. The author believed that hypochondriasis was subconsciously motivated, and expressed surprise at "unexpectedly rapid incomprehensible cures . . . [as a result of] a few psychotherapeutic conversations" in other cases (p. 382). Although the patients were selected for apparent amenability to psychotherapy, only a small proportion recovered or improved with these treatments.

Contemporary therapies tend to address the hypochondriacal fears or false beliefs directly as opposed to searching for unconscious motives. The main strategies employed are in vivo exposure, cognitive-educational strategies, and persuasion. All three methods are plausible and may be used in combination. The most suitable strategy probably depends largely on the patient's psychopathology.

Several authors have advanced the view that exposure is appropriate treatment, based on the belief that hypochondriasis is a disease phobia and is similar to other phobias (Marks 1987). Uncontrolled studies suggest that these strategies are helpful in a substantial proportion of patients (Salkovskis and Warwick 1986; Warwick and Marks 1988). The patient is advised to avoid reassurance through a physician or a spouse. Such reassurance is believed to be similar to escape from a phobic situation or to the rituals of patients with obsessive-compulsive disorder. Such avoidance behavior may yield a temporary relief from anxiety, but it prevents extinction of fear. Persistent exposure to the feared idea and suppression of avoidance will then lead to extinction of the hypochondriacal behavior.

Several other authors have suggested an educational and cognitive approach (Barsky et al. 1988a; Gillespie 1928; House 1989; Kellner 1982; Kulenkampff and Bauer 1960). Patients are offered a cognitive-perceptual model of hypochondriasis. They are taught the principles of selective perception of bodily sensations (Kellner 1982), and somatic symptoms are explained as being analogous to the effects of a radio receiver whose gain is set so high that background static becomes amplified and bothersome (Barksy et al. 1988a). The therapist emphasizes the compatibility of distressing somatic symptoms with excellent physical health and longevity (Kellner 1986). Thus, the patients are given a plausible explanation for their symptoms and fears (House 1989; Salkovskis and Warwick 1986). They are educated about the cycle of the hypochondriacal reaction: fear causes autonomic overactivity that in turn induces or aggravates existing somatic symptoms, thus causing more fear and a vicious cycle (Kellner 1982).

For patients who believe that they suffer from an undetected, perhaps progressive and dangerous disease, it appears to be crucial to their progress to devise methods to convince them that the symptoms are not caused by physical disease and that their beliefs are false. Persuasion and the cognitive-educational approach share several elements. The strategies of psychotherapy with these patients, described in detail elsewhere (Kellner 1986, 1989a), include the following: the building of a therapeutic alliance based on empathy; acceptance of the patient's suffering, the patient's irrational beliefs and demands, and the patient's failure to benefit from reassurance; and respect of the person. Methods of persuasion include explanation, education, retraining of selective perception, and counteraction of iatrogenic false beliefs. Psychotherapeutic "working through" is facilitated by repetition and cognitive exercises.

Pharmacotherapy

There are no controlled drug studies in primary hypochondriasis. In hypochondriacal patients who are anxious or depressed, or in patients in whom there is doubt whether the syndrome is primary or secondary, energetic treatment of coexisting psychiatric disorders needs to be tried. The reason for the efficacy of psychotropic drugs in primary hypochondriasis is unknown—probably the relief from somatic symptoms makes it easier to persuade the patient that he or she is not suffering from a physical disease. The relief of anxiety and depression allows a more robust and resilient attitude toward bodily symptoms.

If all treatments have failed, whether in chronically somatizing patients or in patients with chronic hypochondriacal attitudes, the patient will continue to seek care. Several authors have advocated strategies of dealing with these patients, but there are no empirical studies that allow judgment as to whether some approaches are more advantageous than others. Several authors recommend regularly spaced sessions with the physician (Brown and Vaillant 1981; Busse 1956) for supportive therapy, for the supervision of psychotropic drugs, and for the treatment of coexisting emotional disorders.

Prognosis

Minor and brief hypochondriacal reactions are common (Mayou 1976; Mendel 1889). The duration of somatization in most patients ranges from a few weeks to a few months (Kellner 1963; Thomas 1978), and many of these patients have transient hypochondriacal concerns. Most of these patients recover with routine medical care without any specific treatment directed at their complaints (Thomas 1978). Even some patients with long-standing hypochondriasis will improve with simple treatment, and some even start to improve while waiting for psychiatric treatment (Kellner and Sheffield 1971).

It is possible to define three subgroups of hypochondriasis with different prognoses: 1) *hypochondriacal reaction* (temporary or transitory hypochondriasis) (Ford 1983); 2) *hypochondriacal neurosis*, which can be understood as a reaction of somatization with anxiety, selective attention to bodily sensation (Barsky 1979; Kellner 1986), and a vicious cycle of somatic symptoms, anxiety arousal, and selective attention; and 3) *developmental hypochondriasis* (Ladee 1966), a chronic hypochondriasis with an onset early in life that resembles a personality disorder. The latter subgroup, developmental hypochondriasis, has many features in common with DSM-III-R somatization disorder.

Hypochondriasis can have a fluctuating course. The outcome of hypochondriasis often depends on the nature of the coexisting disorder (Kellner 1983; Ladee 1966; Pilowsky 1968). In several follow-up studies on hypochondriacal patients whose cases were severe enough to be referred to psychiatrists, the number of patients who substantially improved or recovered approached or exceeded 50% (Kellner 1983; Kenyon 1964; Ladee 1966; Pilowsky 1968).

CONCLUSIONS

Anecdotal reports and clinical lore have suggested that somatizing and hypochondriacal patients are difficult to treat. Existing studies, however, suggest that many such patients respond well to appropriate therapy. Effective treatment begins with an empathic understanding and validation of the patient's physical distress. When an underlying mood or anxiety disorder can be detected, treatment of these conditions may resolve somatic symptoms and hypochondriacal fear. Patients with functional somatic symptoms often experience only transient distress that can be reduced with explanation and reassurance. For patients with more severe or persistent forms of somatization, specific interventions may target somatic symptoms, emotional distress, and/or the attitudes and beliefs that undermine coping and amplify somatic distress. Further refinements and recommendations for treatment must await controlled studies of treatment efficacy in somatization.

REFERENCES

American Psychiatric Association: Diagnostic and Statistical Manual of

Mental Disorders, 3rd Edition, Revised. Washington, DC, American Psychiatric Association, 1987

Barsky AJ: Patients who amplify bodily symptoms. Ann Intern Med 91:63–70, 1979

Barsky AJ, Klerman GL: Overview: hypochondriasis, bodily complaints and somatic styles. Am J Psychiatry 140:273–283, 1983

Barsky AJ, Wyshak G: Hypochondriasis and related health attitudes. Psychosomatics 30:412–420, 1989

Barsky AJ, Wyshak G, Klerman GL: Hypochondriasis: an evaluation of the DSM-III criteria in medical outpatients. Arch Gen Psychiatry 43:493–500, 1986

Barsky AJ, Geringer E, Wool CA: A cognitive-educational treatment for hypochondriasis. Gen Hosp Psychiatry 10:322–327, 1988a

Barsky AJ, Goodson JD, Lane RS, et al: The amplification of somatic symptoms. Psychosom Med 50:510–519, 1988b

Bates S, Sjödén PO, Nyrén O: Behavioral treatment of non-ulcer dyspepsia. Scandinavian Journal of Behaviour Therapy 17:155–165, 1988

Biofeedback and tension headache (editorial). Lancet 2:898–899, 1980

Blanchard EB, Schwarz SP, Neff DF, et al: Prediction of outcome from the self-regulatory treatment of irritable bowel syndrome. Behav Res Ther 26:187–190, 1988

Bridges KW, Goldberg DP: Somatic presentation of DSM-III psychiatric disorders in primary care. J Psychosom Res 29:563–569, 1985

Brown HN, Vaillant GE: Hypochondriasis. Arch Intern Med 141:723–726, 1981

Busse EW: The treatment of the chronic complainer. Medical Record and Annals 50:196–200, 1956

Cann PA, Read NW: A disease of the whole gut? in Irritable Bowel Syndrome. Edited by Read NW. New York, Grune & Stratton, 1985, pp 53–66

Cooper CD, Dickinson JR, Adams HB, et al: Interviewer's role-playing and responses to sensory deprivation: a clinical demonstration. Percept Mot Skills 40:291–303, 1975

Coryell W, Norten SG: Briquet's syndrome (somatization disorder) and primary depression: comparison of background and outcome. Compr Psychiatry 22:249–256, 1981

Covi L, Lipman RS, Derogatis LR, et al: Drugs and group psychotherapy in neurotic depression. Am J Psychiatry 131:191–198, 1974

Draspa LJ: Psychological factors in muscular pain. Br J Med Psychol 32:106–116, 1959

Dwan C, Nesbitt J: Group approach to hypochondriasis. Am Fam Physician 18:23, 1978

Ford CV: The Somatizing Disorders: Illness as a Way of Life. New York, Elsevier, 1983

Ford CV, Long KD: Group psychotherapy of somatizing patients. Psychother Psychosom 28:294–304, 1977

Gillespie RD: Hypochondria: its definition, nosology and psychopathology. Guys Hospital Report 8:408–460, 1928

Glass RM, Ulenhuth EH, Kellner R: The value of self-report assessment in studies of anxiety disorders. J Clin Psychopharmacol 7:215–221, 1987

Goldenberg DL, Felson DT, Dinerman H: A randomized, controlled trial of amitriptyline and naproxen in the treatment of patients with fibromyalgia. Arthritis Rheum 29:1371–1377, 1986

Greenbaum DS, Mayle JE, Vanegeren LE, et al: Effects of desipramine on irritable bowel syndrome compared with atropine and placebo. Dig Dis Sci 32:257–266, 1987

Guze SB, Perley MJ: Observations on the natural history of hysteria. Am J Psychiatry 119:960–965, 1963

Holroyd KA, Andrasik F, Westbrook T: Cognitive control of tension headache. Cognitive Therapy and Research 1:121–133, 1977

House A: Hypochondriasis and related disorders. Gen Hosp Psychiatry 11:156–165, 1989

Jessup BA, Neufeld RWJ, Merskey H: Biofeedback therapy for headache and other pain: an evaluative review. Pain 7:225–270, 1979

Kahn RJ, McNair DM, Lipman RS, et al: Imipramine and chlordiazepoxide in depressive and anxiety disorders, II: efficacy in anxious outpatients. Arch Gen Psychiatry 43:79–85, 1986

Kellner R: Neurotic ill health in a general practice on Deeside. Unpublished M.D. Thesis, University of Liverpool, Liverpool, UK, 1963

Kellner R: Neurosis in general practice. Br J Clin Pract 19:681–682, 1965

Kellner R: Psychotherapeutic strategies in hypochondriasis: a clinical study. Am J Psychother 36:146–157, 1982

Kellner R: Prognosis of treated hypochondriasis: a clinical study. Acta Psychiatr Scand 67:69–79, 1983

Kellner R: Somatization and Hypochondriasis. New York, Praeger-Greenwood, 1986

Kellner R: Hypochondriasis and somatization. JAMA 258:2718–2722, 1987

Kellner R: Anxiety, somatic sensations and bodily complaints, in Handbook of Anxiety, Vol. 2: Classification, Etiological Factors and Associated Disturbances. Edited by Noyes R, Roth M, Burrows GD. New York, Elsevier, 1988, pp 213–237

Kellner R: Hypochondriasis and body dysmorphic disorder, in Treatments of Psychiatric Disorders: A Task Force Report of the American Psychiatric Association, Vol 2. Edited by Karasu T and the Task Force on Treatments of Psychiatric Disorders. Washington, DC, American Psychiatric Association, 1989a, pp 2138–2146

Kellner R: Somatization disorder, in Treatments of Psychiatric Disorders: A Task Force Report of the American Psychiatric Association, Vol 2. Edited by Karasu T and the Task Force on Treatments of Psychiatric Disorders. Washington, DC, American Psychiatric Association, 1989b, pp 2166–2171

Kellner R: Somatization: the most costly comorbidity, in Comorbidity of Mood and Anxiety Disorders. Edited by Maser JD, Cloninger CR. Washington, DC, American Psychiatric Press, 1990, pp 239–252

Kellner R, Sheffield BF: The relief of distress following attendance at a clinic. Br J Psychiatry 118:195–198, 1971

Kellner R, Fava GA, Lisansky J, et al: Hypochondriacal fears and beliefs in DSM-III melancholia: changes with amitriptyline. J Affective Disord 10:21–26, 1986

Kellner R, Abbott P, Winslow WW, et al: Fears, beliefs, and attitudes in DSM-III hypochondriasis. J Nerv Ment Dis 175:20–25, 1987

Kellner R, Abbott P, Winslow WW, et al: Anxiety, depression, and somatization in DSM-III hypochondriasis. Psychosomatics 30:57–64, 1989

Kenyon FE: Hypochondriasis: a clinical study. Br J Psychiatry 110:478–488, 1964

Kessel WIN: Psychiatric morbidity in a London general practice. British Journal of Preventive and Social Medicine 14:16–22, 1960

Küchenhoff J: Das hypochondrische Syndrom. Nervenarzt 56:225–236, 1985

Kulenkampff C, Bauer A: Uber das Syndrom der Herzphobie (Schluss). Nervenarzt 31:496–507, 1960

Ladee GA: Hypochondriacal Syndromes. New York, Elsevier, 1966

Lipowski ZJ: Somatization and depression. Psychosomatics 31:13–21, 1990

Mally MA, Ogston WD: Treatment of the "untreatables." Int J Group Psychother 14:369–374, 1964

Marks IM: Fears, Phobias and Rituals: Panic, Anxiety, and Their Disorders. Oxford, Oxford University Press, 1987

Mayou R: The nature of bodily symptoms. Br J Psychiatry 129:55–60, 1976

Mendel E: Hypochondrie beim Weiblichen Geschlecht. Dtsch Med Wochenschr, 1889, pp 205–209

Noyes R Jr, Reich J, Clancy J, et al: Reduction of hypochondriasis with treatment of panic disorder. Br J Psychiatry 149:631–635, 1986

Nuechterlein KH, Holroyd JC: Biofeedback in the treatment of tension headache: current status. Arch Gen Psychiatry 37:866–873, 1980

Okasha A, Ghaleb HA, Sadek A: A double-blind trial for the clinical management of psychogenic headache. Br J Psychiatry 122:181–183, 1973

Ost LG: Applied relaxation: description of an effective coping technique. Scandinavian Journal of Behaviour Therapy 17:83–96, 1988

Patterson JE, Spees DN: Considering the options: a multilevel systemic approach to helping somatizing patients. Family Systems Medicine 6:411–420, 1988

Pilowsky I: The response to treatment in hypochondriacal disorders. Aust NZ J Psychiatry 2:88–94, 1968

Robinson DS, Nies A, Ravaris CL, et al: The monoamine oxidase inhibitor, phenelzine, in the treatment of depressive-anxiety states: a controlled clinical trial. Arch Gen Psychiatry 29:407–413, 1973

Rosenberg S: The relationship of certain personality factors to prognosis in psychotherapy. J Clin Psychol 10:341–345, 1954

Salkovskis PM, Warwick HMC: Morbid preoccupations, health anxiety and reassurance: a cognitive-behavioural approach to hypochondriasis. Behav Res Ther 24:597–602, 1986

Sapira JD: Reassurance therapy. Ann Intern Med 77:603–604, 1972

Scallet A, Cloninger CR, Othmer E: The management of chronic hysteria: a review and double-blind trial of electrosleep and other relaxation methods. J Nerv Ment Dis 37:347–353, 1976

Schonecke OW, Schüffel W: Evaluation of combined pharmacological and psychotherapeutic treatment in patients with functional abdominal disorders. Psychother Psychosom 26:86–92, 1975

Sheehan DV, Ballenger J, Jacobsen G: Treatment of endogenous anxiety with phobic, hysterical, and hypochondriacal symptoms. Arch Gen Psychiatry 37:51–59, 1980

Sjödin I, Svedlund J, Ottosson JO, et al: Controlled study of psychotherapy in chronic peptic ulcer disease. Psychosomatics 27:187–200, 1986

Smith GR, Monson RA, Ray DC: Psychiatric consultation in somatization disorder. N Engl J Med 314:1407–1413, 1986

Stone AR, Frank JD, Hoehn-Saric R, et al: Some situational factors associated with response to psychotherapy. Am J Orthopsychiatry 35:682–687, 1965

Svedlund J, Ottosson J-O, Sjödin I, et al: Controlled study of psychotherapy in irritable bowel syndrome. Lancet 2:589–592, 1983

Thomas KB: The consultation and the therapeutic illusion. Br Med J 1:1327–1328, 1978

Tyrer P: The Role of Bodily Feelings in Anxiety. New York, Oxford University Press, 1976

Uhlenhuth EH, Glass RM, Haberman SJ, et al: Relative sensitivity of clinical measures in trials of anti-anxiety agents, in Quantitative Techniques for the Evaluation of the Behavior of Psychiatric Patients. Edited by Burdock EI, Sudilorsky A, Gershon S. New York, Marcel Dekker, 1982, pp 393–409

Valko RJ: Group therapy for patients with hysteria (Briquet's Disorder). Diseases of the Nervous System 37:484–487, 1976

Warwick HMC, Marks IM: Behavioural treatment of illness phobia and hypochondriasis: a pilot study of 17 cases. Br J Psychiatry 152:239–241, 1988

Wessely S, David A, Butler S, et al: Management of chronic (post-viral) fatigue syndrome. J R Coll Gen Pract 39:26–29, 1989

Whorwell PJ, Prior A, Faragher ER: Controlled trial of hypnotherapy in the treatment of severe refractory irritable-bowel syndrome. Lancet 2:1232–1234, 1984

Yalom ID: Theory and Practice of Group Psychotherapy. New York, Basic Books, 1970

Yunus MB, Masi AT: Association of primary fibromyalgia syndrome (PFS) with stress-related syndromes. Abstract of presentation at the 50th annual meeting of the American Rheumatism Association, and the 21st annual meeting of the Arthritis Health Professions Association, June 1986

Chapter 9

Somatization in Cultural and Historical Perspective

Horacio Fabrega, Jr., M.D.

T he term *somatization* describes the presentation of medical-psychological and especially psychiatric problems in terms of bodily symptoms and distress (Barsky and Klerman 1983; Ford 1986; Kellner 1986; Lipowski 1988). The existence of different concepts of somatization has recently been emphasized (Kirmayer 1984). Regardless of whether it functions as displaced psychosocial distress, a variation of major depressive or anxiety disorders, or preoccupation and worry about physical illness and well-being, somatization connotes psychiatric morbidity and the illusion of general medical morbidity.

In this chapter the concept of somatization is analyzed in cultural and historical perspective. First, assumptions implicit in the current use of the concept of somatization are discussed with the aim of making clear the underlying Western medical perspective. Second, the concept is examined in relation to knowledge from the fields of medical anthropology and the early history of medicine, in order to compare how somatization and related phenomena pertaining to health, illness, and adaptation are handled in different medical systems. Finally, developments in the modern history of medicine that have conditioned and shaped the concept of somatization and its supporting theory are outlined and discussed.

THE DUALISTIC EPISTEMOLOGY OF WESTERN MEDICINE

The concept of somatization owes its rationale to a dualistic epistemology that is deeply embedded in the history of European medical theory and practice. This epistemology references a model of *illness*, that is, how a person behaves and should behave in the context of specific, measurable *disease* changes in the body. The model encompasses reports of pain, bodily experience, and physiological dysfunction as well as appropriate degrees and forms of worry, modes of social role functioning, and medical care seeking. This model of illness allows one to specify that a person's responses to physiological or anatomical changes constitute deviations from expected norms. It is when such responses deviate from cultural norms that physicians bring into play the concept of somatization.

The dualistic epistemology of Western medicine embodies a theory of disease that is both functional and ontological. The theory is "functional" in that elaborate physiological and chemical processes are held to account for disease.[1] These processes are influenced by characteristics of the individual: genetics, social background, and current life habits realize a unique disease picture. At the same time, the theory is ontological, holding that diseases have an existence and identity of their own. This means diseases are like objects with a distinctive developmental unfolding or natural history that is independent of the person. The notions of a functional and ontological approach to disease are used comparatively below.

Western medicine postulates a correspondence and association between illness (as subjective distress) and disease (as objectively verifiable organic disturbance) (Jennings 1986). Persons whose bodies are not altered or diseased should demonstrate no illness, and those persons who do display such distress should be diseased. While correspondence might mean only correlation—which does not imply causation or directionality—the logic of biomedicine often assumes a directionality with disease leading to illness. Implicit in applications of biomedical theory, then, is a form of determinism, if not reductionism, that assigns priority to the phenomena of disease.

The close link between illness and disease can be seen as a result both of the evolution of science and of the state's ability to legitimate and authenticate the status of disability (Stone 1984). Strict application of the verification system underlying diagnosis leads to claims—for example, "some ill persons are not diseased"—that imply dissimulation and malingering. Except in situations requiring legal determinations of disability, such claims are usually not made for several reasons. One involves the idea that persons are ordinarily held to be authentic and credible social beings. To preserve this credibility, continued claims of illness in the absence of disease are explained in terms of Western psychological ideas about unconscious mental phenomena, psychosomatic mediation, and, more recently, somatization. In addition, given an appreciation of the limitations of biomedi-

---

[1]This philosophical use of the term functional as *explanation in terms of function or process* differs from its conventional medical use to refer to disturbances with no detectable organic cause.

cal knowledge and the quandaries of mind-body correspondence, a claim of dissimulation or malingering is often both logically and psychologically unfounded. Political and economic factors tied to the practice of medicine in a market economy contribute to the medical appropriation of persons claiming illness (even without identifiable organic disease) as really being sick, requiring treatment, and, hence, constituting legitimate consumers of medical care. Finally, biological and social science theories of adaptation and general systems theory underscore the role of stress in producing illness. Persons who claim illness but are not diseased may be viewed as showing the effects of social maladaptation beyond their control, thus legitimating their claims as medically compromised.

CONCEPTS OF SOMATIZATION AND ELEMENTARY MEDICAL SYSTEMS

Studies in medical anthropology have made abundantly clear the important role played by illness and medical care in the social life of communities (Fabrega 1972; Kleinman 1980; Scott 1963; Young 1976). Episodes of illness constitute or reflect social, religious, political, and moral crises. Illness distress and illness behavior, in the light of the explanatory models prevalent in the society, are seen to reflect relations with the ancestors, the breaking of social taboos, and political rivalries. The symbols used to explain and treat illness use the somatic components of illness as concrete markers of the actions of causal agents. Treatment involves social and political rituals tied to body changes, including symptoms of bodily dysfunction, bodily products, and body fluids. The somatic concomitants of illness as well as its social role are linked to symbols with ecological, social, and cultural significance within the society (Hughes 1968).

The possibility of illness is a worrisome preoccupation because disabling illness is common, seriously compromising the ability of highly integrated groups to subsist and reproduce. Researchers have shown the wide-ranging roles that conversations about the body and illness play in defining states of self and in establishing social networks. These "somatic dialogues" are not limited exclusively to episodes of illness but serve to communicate distress and worry over a host of social and existential happenings that are thereby socially and culturally somatized.

All of the preceding implies that the language of the body plays a central anchoring role in the cultural dynamics of illness and healing in elementary societies. Features of the language of the body correspond to (or connect with) diverse phenomena including the self, the social, the natural, and the supernatural—all of which make up the behavioral environment of the community. In this setting, illness is a social drama. If a "correspondence" linked to body changes could be said to exist, it would be shown to connect not to an individual mind but to phenomena that at once embrace and transcend the individual.

In elementary societies, individuals are not seen as discrete, willful, autonomous agents comprised of minds and bodies that operate like (dualistic) machines (Schweder and Bourne 1982). Validation of illness does not involve appeals to biological technologies, but remains anchored to individual perceptions of illness. Illness is a social affair because it affects the person's immediate group, and treatment involves the members of this group. The causes of illness—but not its reality—may be problematic and negotiated along social, moral, and political lines. The system of medicine appropriates, validates, and distributes causal attributions so as to resolve the social burdens linked to illness in an optimal way (Fabrega 1976; Press 1980). This system, however, does not invalidate illnesses, nor does it morally discredit sick persons, by labeling certain illness as less than fully authentic or as psychiatric. The idea that an illness is ontologically different or less authentic because it represents a "mere displacement" onto the somatic sphere has no warrant in the societies in question.

Distinctions between psychiatric and nonpsychiatric illnesses are not prevalent in elementary societies. In Anglo-American societies, psychiatric illnesses and diseases are associated with a special ontology and epistemology (e.g., the mind or brain as the source of psychopathological symptoms) and with discrediting social responses (psychiatric stigma). Such distinctions are not found in elementary societies. Instead, one finds a form of stigma that can attach to any (usually protracted) illness depending on its putative etiology and social interpretation (e.g., witchcraft or ancestor punishment). Psychiatric illnesses are not characteristically given a negative interpretation, nor are special types of illnesses labeled differently so as to link with the psychiatric and, hence, discredit or weaken the authenticity of persons who display them.

In summary, somatization concepts, with their implications of mind-body dualism, have no meaning and application in the systems of medicine of elementary societies. The dualistic epistemology of biomedicine and the concept of somatization that it makes necessary seem to require an ontological view of disease, a social system wherein individualistic agents bear the responsibility and social consequences of illness, a biological mode of verification, and a medical and political system ready to use the resultant implication that the sick individual "somatizer" is less than fully authentic or is ill in a different way from others.

CONCEPTS OF SOMATIZATION IN AN INDIAN MEDICAL CONTEXT

An ontological distinction between mental and physical disease would appear to be crucial in establishing a typology within which certain deviant forms of distress could be characterized as somatization. Many traditional systems of medicine do not provide such ontological distinctions. For example, the idea of separate disease entities, each having distinctive causes, mechanisms, symptom profiles, treatments, and prognoses, did not gain dominance in India. The theory of Ayurvedic medicine is powerfully unitary and functional in nature and does not distinguish ontologically among types or nature of medical disease.

The traditional theory and practice of medicine developed in India constitutes one of mankind's most comprehensive and elaborated systems of knowledge (Basham 1976; Kutumbiah 1969; Leslie 1976). The period of the rise of the great classical medical schools and the writings of the great physicians (600 B.C.–200 A.D.) involved the refinement of anatomy, physiology, pathophysiology, and therapeutics. The theory of medicine was grounded in the main doctrines of the schools of philosophy known as the Nyàya-Vaisesika. In the writings of Charaka, key philosophical concepts pertaining to the nature of things in the world and the basic categories and their modes of operating, were taken over—and, in some instances, modified—to structure medical knowledge and practice.

The resulting theory of Ayurvedic medicine is anchored in the elements of the cosmos that are believed to have their microsomic counterparts in the organism. Five basic constituents that account for the permanence and functioning of the body are said to exist. The doctrine of the three *dosas* occupies a central role in the theory of illness, symptom development, and therapeutics. The dosas, which exist in different forms, are described as faults or vitiators of the body constituents and are subject to excess or diminished activity. They can be disturbed singly or in combination, thus both affecting physiological well-being and contributing to the temperament and behavior of a person.

Disease is defined as involving a disharmony among the bodily constituents and/or their excess or deficient amounts and activity. Filliozat (1969, p. 82) has pointed out that "not every kind of excess or deficiency of the [body constituents] produces a disequilibrium [or disease]: it is only when such deficiency or excess produces affections of the body that it is so called. Slight variations of the due proportions [or constituents] cannot be called [disease or disharmony] unless accompanied by . . . external symptoms." Similarly, Filliozat notes, "each of the so-called diseases of Indian medicine was nothing but a vague symptom complex which, upon the slightest deviation from its supposed type, dissolved, to reappear in a number of fresh categories" (p. 98). Diseases or symptoms, then, can be primary or can function as causes or premonitory evidence of other diseases (i.e., symptoms and symptom complexes). Filliozat further points out: "Sometimes one symptom belongs to many diseases, also one symptom may belong to one disease. Many symptoms again are manifested by one disease, also many symptoms are manifested by many diseases" (pp. 98–99). Each symptom is given attention in its own right and in relation to others, with respect to underlying etiology, pathogenesis, course, duration, and response to treatment. Importantly, in the doctrine of the dosas, all symptoms are examined and explained in terms of bodily constituents. The schema of causes and influences that the latter are subject to, span climate, weather, food intake, physical activity, psychological activity, and emotional phenomena.

The causes, pathogenesis, and manifestations of illness (i.e., symptoms), diagnosis, treatment, and even the ascertainment of prognosis thus all encompass physical, physiological, and mental phenomena. In other words, every facet of illness and disease can involve phenomena that cross the mind-body duality of the West. Obeyesekere (1977) indicates that "in the classical theories of Susruta and Caraka, the major cause of mental malfunction is the upsetting of the humors [the dosas], as in all diseases" (p. 159). These can be disturbed by a variety of factors, and the "types of madness" are said to be several. Premonitory symptoms of madness span our psychological, neurological, and visceral physiological domains. Obeyesekere continues: "Note that the same causes can produce imbalance and bring about diseases which *do not* affect the mind. . . . Basically, the principle of cure is the same in all diseases: the upset humor [dosa] has to be controlled by ingredients that have the right counteractive properties . . . [and] similar causes can produce different diseases: the crucial fact again is the *manner* in which the intervening humors are affected. . . . Ayurveda recognizes strictly psychosomatic illness, though they do not receive conceptual formulation. . . . Emotional conditions like sorrow or excitement cannot only produce madness . . . [but also] through a radically different effect on the dosas (humors), diseases which have nothing to do with mind, but are entirely organic or physical" (p. 159). These generalizations also apply to principles of therapeutics, since the same therapies can be used for different illnesses.

Because there exists one system of physiology to explain all illnesses and the system is rooted in the report of illness (i.e., symptoms), it follows that ideas of somatization, as phenomena of illness that are different, excessive, displaced, or unrelated to disease, have no warrant in Ayurvedic medicine. Any and all illness-distress phenomena have to be accorded equal weight, since there does not exist an epistemology, much less a technology, that serves to equate mind and behavior with anatomy and physiology or to validate illness independent of its report. Illness and disease thus are not logically disconnected categories as they are in modern biomedicine. Indeed, bodily, mental, and spiritual well-being and moral identity all flow out of, and are made sense of, in terms of a comprehensive system that embraces and gives exquisite attention to bodily experience and function.

CONCEPTS OF SOMATIZATION IN A CHINESE MEDICAL CONTEXT

Medicine as a theory of knowledge, a system of practice, and an institution of society has an important textual tradition in Chinese societies dating back before the first millennium B.C. (Gwei-Djewn and Needham 1980; Hume 1975; Porkert and Illman 1982; Unschuld 1983, 1985a, 1985b; Yanchi 1988). Up until the 20th century, medicine in China relied on a number of theories identified with philosophical and ethical-religious schools including Taoism, Buddhism, and Confucianism. Concepts and explanatory models from each of these schools have been applied to illness and, together with their therapeutic rationales, modified, expanded, and refined over time.

In the "medicine of systematic correspondence" that has occupied a very prominent place in Chinese medicine, the body is seen as vulnerable to attack by outside agencies. Through its own defenses, the body is able to ward off such attacks. Health problems can also stem from "antagonisms" or disturbances among the body's internal components. Functional units of the body are seen as ordinarily mutually interdependent, but under conditions of "weakness" in any one of them, they become vulnerable to harmful influences. The evil influences responsible for disease are not limited to demons, but include "empirically visible influences and emanations" (Unschuld 1985a, p. 68) that require man to live in harmony with phenomena of the natural world in order to maintain an inner bodily harmony that constitutes freedom from illness. Wind and rain were related to the activities of the supreme celestial spirit who could occupy any of the eight principal locations of the compass in a distinctive order and at specific times. The direction of the wind on those dates provided clues to disease etiology. Unschuld (1985a) points out the importance of "the inevitability, of the external determination of illness as soon as someone is struck by a depletion-wind" (p. 69). Yet, as Unschuld notes, it was also held that it is "the physiological condition of the organism that creates the disposition for possible injury by wind" (p. 70), in particular those occasioned by the phase of life of the person, the changing phases of the moon, and the kind of adaptation during critical phases of life.

Eleven isolated vessels in the body were held to contain vital material in circulation or movement. Twelve connecting conduits served as channels for the circulation of substance between these vessels. In illness this constant natural flow could slow down, congeal, and settle in or outside the vessels. The conduit vessels themselves came to be associated with organs of the body that were classified with respect to Yin and Yang qualities—opposite but complementary forces that ceaselessly rise and fall. Life was believed to depend on innate primordial *ch'i* influences, which could be depleted through wasteful expenditure, and on ch'i influences produced inside by the organism. Health required the intake of external influences in their proper proportions to balance the loss of innate ones, and the transport of material to the various organs through the transportation channels. Harmonious circulation, with the avoidance of "depletions" and "repletions" in the organs and obstructions in the vessels, was the fundamental idea explaining bodily function and health.

Porkert and Illman (1982) have lucidly described the central importance of the function circle of the heart in Chinese medicine. It and its product or emanation (*shen*) are seen as the essence of all vital activity in the body and are responsible for the expressions of a person's individuality, including consciousness, concentration, reasoning, and organized social action. Disturbances in this function circle are said to be associated with a disintegration of the coherence of the personality, cognitive clarity, and organized behavior. If prolonged and untreated, this disturbance can lead to insanity, epilepsy, or other physiological symptoms. This linking of the heart, to us quintessentially a bodily or organic entity, with behavioral phenomena we think of as mental, underscores the holism implicit in Chinese medicine. It rationalizes methods of psychodiagnosis and psychotherapeutic treatment *for all disease*—not just for our mental ones.

In ancient Chinese medicine, disturbance of bodily function was believed to manifest outwardly in the form of symptoms, and these, when properly analyzed, could reveal the nature of illness that involved an imbalance of some sort. Yanchi (1988, p. 18) describes the nature of this imbalance:

> This essential imbalance is . . . the so-called *symptom complex . . .* [and] Chinese medicine does not distinguish different diseases: it differentiates symptom complexes . . . [that are] different from a symptom. Symptoms are manifestations [of disordered physiology, behavior, and mentation]. A symptom-complex is a complete summarization of the functioning of the body at a particular stage of the illness . . . [which] includes symptoms [that are seen as links to] a basic imbalance in the functioning of the body.

It should be clear that the ideas of a psychiatric disease or illness have little meaning in this system of medicine. Although it is possible to identify some elements of Western psychiatric illness in traditional texts, these are not represented as being equivalent to our nosological entities. That is to say, features of Western psychiatric illness are included (e.g., wandering, restlessness, seeing demons) but are seen as components of "symptom complexes" that are large-scale physiological imbalances:

> When diagnosis is based on differentiating symptom complexes, several . . . [of these] may account for a condition that in Western medicine is viewed as a single disease. On the other hand, the same symptom complex can appear in a variety of different diseases at some stage in their development. Since treatment follows diagnosis, a single disease . . . may be treated by different methods, and different diseases may be treated by the same method. (Yanchi 1988, p. 19)

In this system of medicine, illness symptoms are part of what ails the patient and what propels him or her to seek treatment. The continued presence of symptoms, in the light of other external manifestations reflecting bodily function and cosmic relatedness, recommends the treatment.

Traditional Chinese medicine never developed a model of how illness is structured in relation to independent organic events that could serve both to establish and to validate the presence of disease. Nor did it develop an ontological view of disease in which different illnesses could be characterized as more or less authentic. Consequently, in classical Chinese medicine the idea of somatization as exaggerated, excessive, displaced, or peculiarly manufactured bodily symptoms simply does not exist.

CONCEPTS OF SOMATIZATION IN THE EARLY EUROPEAN CONTEXT

The Euro-Mediterranean tradition of medicine dominated the thinking of the academic physicians of Western Europe until approximately the 16th century (Lloyd 1979; Phillips 1973; Saunders 1963; Scarborough 1969; Temkin 1973). It also had a preponderant influence on medieval Islamic medicine (Ullman 1978). In this tradition, the Hippocratic corpus and the writings of Galen were preeminent. The ideas of this tradition are generally well known and do not require detailed review or discussion.

Greek medicine held a functional view of diseases as disturbances in an elaborate physiology centered on the four humors and the pneuma (Nutton 1983; Temkin 1963). Attributes of the person and his or her biography uniquely determined pathology. Galenic physiology addressed disease symptomatology, descriptions of pain, and bodily dysfunction, as well as the prevention of illness and, indeed, the maintenance of health. The theory of illness and health included concepts and explanations pertaining to the weather, climate, seasons of the year, diet, exercise, and hygiene. The unity of the mental and the bodily, conceptualized as personal patterns of the humors and pneuma, and the relationship of these patterns to environmental factors, were cornerstones of the Hippocratic and Galenic theories. Hinted at in the former, and explicit and fully developed in the latter, were ideas pertaining to psychological types (the choleric and phlegmatic temperaments, etc.) and their contribution to health and illness.

To a much less developed extent, Greek and Hellenistic medicine also reflects a view of diseases as distinct entities (Nutton 1983; Temkin 1963). Rooted in definitions that gave a central role to both bodily and mental symptoms, the Greeks developed a typology that included disease entities that recurred and that had a putative universality transcending space and time. Their disease entities can in some instances be equated with our general medical (e.g., tuberculosis, malaria) and psychiatric (e.g., delirium, psychoses, hysteria) diseases. However, although this rudimentary ontological view was evident, and with it the stipulation of types with their own causes and natural histories (e.g., the notion of "seeds" of disease), the functional view of disease was dominant in medical theory and practice. Moreover, inconsistencies and dilemmas created by the ontological view versus the functional view were never really confronted, much less resolved, in Greek medicine.

In contrast to the writings that comprise Chinese and Indian medicine, any contemporary Western physician who reads the writings of Greek physicians has little difficulty identifying with their perspective (Grmek 1989). The Greeks anticipated our current medical logic that emphasizes the role of environment and diet in causing alterations in bodily physiology that in turn manifest as discrete symptoms. The vividness and clarity of descriptions of symptoms are consistent with their use in distinguishing discrete diseases. Although our mental and physical diseases are recognizable in Greek writings, they are all included in general medical works. Regardless of the type of manifestation, diseases were given a bodily physiological explanation in terms of the humors (Jackson 1969). Mental and psychiatric conditions then had no separate status in causality, physiology, or treatment regimen. Although not stigmatized within the medical tradition itself, behaviors corresponding to our mental illness did carry a stigma in social settings (Milns 1986; Rosen 1968).

The importance of bodily symptoms as hallmarks of disease processes and the role played by the physiological and ontological approaches are factors that led to the creation of hysteria as a bona fide Greek "disease" (Veith 1965). However, this disease was not qualified as specious or differentiated from others with respect to its essential nature. An emerging ontological view of disease and the description of entities like hysteria, hypochondria, and certain varieties of melancholia may be considered as providing the semantic roots for our concepts of somatization. It is important to stress that these terms designated illness states consisting of somatic problems suffused with behavioral ones, that these were accorded realities no different from other diseases, and that individuals so diagnosed were not viewed as anomalous or as posing a special problem to physicians. Furthermore, all of these illnesses included somatic symptoms that were chronic in nature, and all were accorded an ontology that was as palpable and real—indeed, equivalent to—madness or insanity. It is problematic to equate such illnesses with contemporary somatization problems. One can speculate that some examples subsumed under the rubric of hysteria (and probably also hypochondria and melancholia) included conditions associated with organic pathology now named and explained differently (Veith 1965). It is, however, reasonable to assume that many did not and arose from mechanisms still unclear. The important point is that such conditions were accorded equal reality in nosologies that mainly reflected a functional view of disease.

In summary, some of the illness problems captured by our concepts of somatization may have been accorded a distinct identity in the classical, Hellenistic, and medieval eras. One could even infer that "somatization disorders" were present in an embryonic form in early Western systems of medicine. However, they were not accorded a different status from other general illnesses. Experience of illness certified disease, and any and all forms of distress received validity in the nosology.

SOMATIZATION IN THE MODERN EUROPEAN MEDICAL CONTEXT

My aim here is to briefly survey two recent historical trends that have contributed to concepts of somatization in Western medicine. One trend, evident early in the Euro-Mediterranean tradition of medicine, authenticates somatization as a distinct medical problem. The other trend, clearly evident by the 17th century, integrates somatization with mental or psychiatric phenomena.

Dualism was prominent in the evolution of psychiatry as a medical and academic discipline during the 19th century. Studies of psychiatric illness concentrated on "madness" and drew attention to intellectual factors involving cognition, rationality, and so forth (Altschule 1976; Berrios 1984, 1987, 1988). A review of theoretical writings from this time reveals an emphasis on psychological ("moral") factors, both as causing disorders and, in the ontological sense, as constituting the phenomena of illness. At the same time, "somaticists"—following the work of Gall—viewed psychiatric phenomena as consequences of cerebral disease and searched for brain lesions.

In both of these lines of theoretical writing, one finds a shared point of view regarding the nature of psychopathology. Psychiatric disorders were accorded a special status that set psychiatry apart from neurology. Even in the writings of Griesinger one notes, despite pleas for the search for the cerebral localization of mental diseases and symptoms, a belief that not all specific cerebral lesions of disease produced mental symptoms—he thought that the cerebral disorders with diffuse pathology were most likely to do so (Ackernecht 1959). Moreover, Griesinger's theory of psychiatric diseases, despite its obvious somatic basis, took into account a host of psychological influences. Parenthetically, Griesinger also gave attention to the clinical changes seen in melancholia and hypochondriasis that he viewed as involving errors in individuals' judgment or perception of their own health to which other psychological factors might contribute. In summary, in the writings of the psychiatrists of the 19th century, one finds an emphasis on specific organic pathology producing mental symptoms that were also influenced by psychological factors. The theme of the interplay between bodily and mental factors came to be applied to somatization problems that were claimed for psychiatry.

A second line of development that contributed to the concept of somatization as a psychiatric disorder began squarely in general academic medicine with the evolution of the concept of *neurosis*

(Bowman 1975; Lopez-Piñero 1983). It is generally regarded that William Cullen (1710–1790) coined the term *neurosis* to refer to nervous force or energy (Jackson 1972). "Energy" was used as an explanatory concept to account for the genesis of forms of nervous disease and its manifestations that had concerned physicians as far back as Sydenham (see also Boss 1979; Brain 1963; Risse 1988).

In the 17th-century mechanistic medical tradition, the nervous system came to play a dominant role in reductionistic explanations of disease. Illnesses otherwise glossed as hysterical, hypochondriacal, or melancholic came to be equated with nervous changes of various types—for example, nervous system weakness, irritation, spasms, and faulty reflexes. In an era when ideas of specific causation, treatment, and neuroanatomical localization were poorly developed, much of the nomenclature and nosology in medicine and neurology was functional in nature. Hence, concepts of nervous force, nervous energy or neurosis played crucial roles in theory and practice, operating in a symbolic way—much like the animal spirits of the Galenic tradition—to explain the pathophysiology of disease.

Many medical, neurological, and psychiatric illnesses were classified as "neuroses." Physicians adopting this perspective were academics of mainstream general medicine and did not, as a rule, give any special attention to traditional psychiatric illnesses involving madness or insanity. Psychiatry at this time was poorly differentiated. Political and economic developments that culminated in institutionalization, with the attendant opportunities for the examination and study of insane persons, did not occur until a generation later. By the end of the 19th century, the list of "neuroses" mainly involved hysteria, hypochondria, and neurasthenia, which were increasingly seen as psychological conditions. Whereas the earlier trend was to stress the organic nature of psychological or mental conditions, this new line of thinking—originating in general medicine and continuing on through the modern ideas of Janet and Freud—converted what had been thought of as organic conditions into psychological ones.

Integral to these 19th-century developments was a consolidation of the modern concept of disease (Cohen 1961; Hudson 1983; Kraupl-Taylor 1980, 1982; Rather 1959). The early emphasis of Paracelsus and van Helmont on disease "seeds" and unique developmental patterns (see Pagel 1972; Pagel and Winder 1968) was augmented by the clinico-anatomical method and the findings of microbiology to reinforce the view of disease as having a distinct ontology. Initially, disease was thought to be constituted in anatomic lesions, later in physiological lesions, and, ultimately, in "psychological lesions," as in the neuroses.

There was parallel development in the semiology of disease. Signs were no longer seen as symbolic of underlying disease but as *external manifestations* of the disease. Clinical descriptions emphasized public and objective parameters such as color, odor, sound, consistency, temperature, and physical dimensions. This trend towards objectification was linked to the rise in medical diagnostic technology (Foucault 1973; Reiser 1978). Eventually, this approach influenced the semiology of psychopathology and mental disease (Berrios 1984, 1988). The mind and behavior were handled as quasiphysical things, parceled up into sensations, perceptions, ideas, beliefs, judgments, feelings, and self-awareness as though each of these functions had an objective anatomical brain locus or representation. Abnormalities in these spheres were then signs of mental or brain diseases. Our terminology of clinical phenomenology and descriptive psychopathology is an outgrowth of these 19th-century developments.

All of these approaches to the study of general medical and mental diseases are important with respect to somatization, since they came to be applied to states such as stupor, fatigue, asthenia, adynamia, and irritability, which eventually came to be seen as hallmarks of the neuroses, hysteria, hypochondriasis, and neurasthenia (Berrios 1981, 1990). Debates as to the physical versus mental nature of fatigue, as in neurasthenia or psychasthenia, focused the brain-behavior or body-mind problem on how to account for somatized problems.

The psychiatric and general medical lines of evolution reviewed here have largely fused during the 20th century. The influences of psychoanalysis and phenomenology heightened the emphasis on the emotional and mental aspects of all psychiatric illness, including somatization. In association with developments in psychophysiology and behavioral medicine, this increased emphasis has allowed the formulation of a postulate of a correspondence and association between illness and disease (or mind and body) and a distinctive cultural model of illness distress and illness behavior.

SUMMARY AND CONCLUSIONS

Phenomena that today are explained as somatization have a long history in Western medicine, and the very concepts used to explain them are rooted in cultural and medical epistemologies of antiquity. In early Western medicine, analogues of somatization disorders such as hysteria and hypochondria were not accorded a different status from other diseases that today we term medical, neurological, or psychiatric. Associated with the Euro-Mediterranean medical typology was a functional theory of illness that focused on the individual's physiology, pathology, and psychology in the light of personal biography and contingent factors. The social system in which these medical ideas operated drew emphasis to individual autonomy. The person came to be seen as responsible for disease and as the bearer of its burdens and qualifications. In the 16th century, the modern ontological view of disease became better articulated. In succeeding centuries, ideas of nervous mechanisms gained prominence in explanations of the conditions we explain with reference to somatization. Under the combined impact of the clinico-anatomical method of the 19th century, the science of semiology and descriptive psychopathology, developments in general pathology and neuropathology, and the elaboration of psychological models of hysteria and neurasthenia, many diseases that had been viewed as organic nervous conditions came to be seen as psychological in nature. Bodily experience was increasingly linked to features of mental functioning and emotional well-being. At the same time, the notion that mental conflicts can produce bodily symptoms has conferred the social stigma of psychiatric labeling on persons with a somatization disorder.

In many non-Western societies, a functional view of disease has dominated. In elementary societies, this view encompasses the individual in his or her (ethno)physiological and (ethno)psychological uniqueness, but this view is also social, religious, and political. However, native theories of illness tend to be relatively unelaborated with respect to pathology and physiology. In societies where the "great traditions of medicine" are dominant, theories of great complexity are found. The functional view, then, gives rise to highly elaborated notions about physiology, pathology, and psychology, encompassing ecological and moral aspects as well. However, in most non-Western systems of medicine, an ontological view of disease never achieved dominance. Hence no basis existed for typing persons with disease labels that carry unique identities. Moreover, a system of external validation of illness never materialized. Symptoms and symptom complexes constituted the basic data of medicine. Because a holistic somatopsychic integration existed in the theory of pathology and physiology, few warrants were present for the differential ontology and valuation of disease entities. Finally, the cultures of the societies in question tend not to be individualistic but sociocentric. The family and immediate group connect to the person, and illness partakes of this sociocentric quality. Any moral valuations that may attach to distinct disease labels are not likely to produce as much social discrediting and personal stigma, since diseases do not exclusively map onto individuals, but connect with the family and group and embrace ongoing social events. Thus, the unique social implications that the concepts of somatization portend for sick persons are not found fully elaborated in non-Western settings.

REFERENCES

Ackernecht EH: A Short History of Psychiatry. London, Hafner, 1959

Altschule MD: Historical perspective—evolution of the concept of schizophrenia, in The Biology of the Schizophrenic Process. Edited by Wolf S, Berle BB. New York, Plenum, 1976, pp 1–15

Barsky AJ, Klerman GL: Overview: hypochondriasis, bodily complaints, and somatic styles. Am J Psychiatry 140:273–283, 1983

Basham AL: The practice of medicine in ancient and medieval India, in Asian Medical Systems. Edited by Leslie C. Berkeley, CA, University of California Press, 1976, pp 18–43

Berrios GE: Stupor: a conceptual history. Psychol Med 11:677–688, 1981

Berrios GE: Descriptive psychopathology: conceptual and historical aspects. Psychol Med 14:303–313, 1984

Berrios GE: Historical aspects of psychoses: 19th century issues. Br Med Bull 43:484–498, 1987

Berrios GE: Historical background to abnormal psychology, in Adult Abnormal Psychology. Edited by Miller E, Cooper PJ. Edinburgh, Churchill Livingston, 1988, pp 26–51

Berrios GE: Feelings of fatigue and psychopathology: a conceptual history. Compr Psychiatry 31:140–151, 1990

Boss JMN: The seventeenth-century transformation of the hysteric affection, and Sydenham's Baconian medicine. Psychol Med 9:221–234, 1979

Bowman LA: William Cullen (1710–90) and the primacy of the nervous system. Unpublished doctoral dissertation, Indiana University, Bloomington, IN, 1975

Brain L: The concept of hysteria in the time of William Harvey. Proceedings of the Royal Society of Medicine 56:317–324, 1963

Cohen H: The evolution of the concept of disease, in Concepts of Medicine. Edited by Lush B. New York, Pergamon, 1961, pp 159–169

Fabrega H: Medical anthropology, in Biennial Review of Anthropology. Edited by Siegel BJ. Stanford, CA, Stanford University Press, 1972, pp 167–229

Fabrega H: The function of medical systems: a logical analysis. Perspect Biol Med 20:108–119, 1976

Filliozat J: The Classical Doctrine of Indian Medicine. Delhi, Munshiram Manoharial, 1969

Ford CV: The somatizing disorders. Psychosomatics 27:327–337, 1986

Foucault M: The Birth of the Clinic. New York, Random House, 1973

Grmek MD: Diseases in the Ancient Greek World. Baltimore, MD, Johns Hopkins University Press, 1989

Gwei-Djewn L, Needham J: Celestial Lancets: A History and Rationale of Acupuncture and Moxa. Cambridge, UK, Cambridge University Press, 1980

Hudson RP: Disease and Its Control: The Shaping of Modern Thought. Westport, CT, Greenwood Press, 1983

Hughes CC: Ethnomedicine, in International Encyclopedia of the Social Sciences. New York, Macmillan, 1968

Hume E: The Chinese Way in Medicine. Westport, CT, Hyperion Press, 1975

Jackson SW: Galen—on mental disorders. J Hist Behav Sci 5:365–384, 1969

Jackson SW: Force and kindred notions in eighteenth-century neurophysiology and medical psychology. Bull Hist Med 44:539–554, 1972

Jennings D: The confusion between disease and illness in clinical medicine. Can Med Assoc J 135:865–870, 1986

Kellner RA: Somatization and Hypochondriasis. New York, Praeger, 1986

Kirmayer LJ: Culture, affect and somatization. Transcultural Psychiatric Research Review 21:159–188, 1984

Kleinman AM: Patients and Healers in the Context of Culture. Berkeley, CA, University of California Press, 1980

Kraupl-Taylor K: The concepts of disease. Psychol Med 10:419–424, 1980

Kraupl-Taylor K: Sydenham's disease entities. Psychol Med 12:243–250, 1982

Kutumbiah P: Ancient Indian Medicine, Revised Edition. Bombay, Orient Longman, 1969

Leslie C: Asian Medical Systems. Berkeley, CA, University of California Press, 1976

Lipowski ZJ: Somatization: the concept and its clinical application. Am J Psychiatry 145:1358–1368, 1988

Lloyd GER: Magic, Reason and Experience. Cambridge, UK, Cambridge University Press, 1979

Lopez-Piñero JM: Historical Origins of the Concept of Neurosis. Cambridge, UK, Cambridge University Press, 1983

Milns RD: Attitudes towards mental illness in antiquity. Aust N Z J Psychiatry 20:454–462, 1986

Nutton V: The seeds of disease: an exploration of contagion and infection from the Greeks to the Renaissance. Med Hist 27:1–34, 1983

Obeyesekere G: The theory and practice of psychological medicine in the Ayurvedic tradition. Cult Med Psychiatry 1:155–181, 1977

Pagel W: Van Helmont's concept of disease—to be or not to be? The influence of Paracelsus. Bull Hist Med 46:419–454, 1972

Pagel W, Winder M: Harvey and the "modern" concept of disease. Bull Hist Med 42:496–509, 1968

Phillips EK: Greek Medicine. London, Thames and Hudson, 1973

Porkert M, Illman C: Chinese Medicine. New York, William Morrow, 1982

Press I: Problems in the definition and classification of medical systems. Soc Sci Med 148:45–47, 1980

Rather LJ: Towards a philosophical study of the idea of disease, in The Historical Development of Physiological Thought. Edited by Brooks CM, Cranefield PF. New York, Hafner, 1959, pp 351–373

Reiser SJ: Medicine and the Reign of Technology. New York, Cambridge University Press, 1978

Risse GB: Hysteria at the Edinburgh infirmary: the construction and treatment of a disease, 1770–1800. Med Hist 32:1–22, 1988

Rosen G: Madness in Society. Chicago, IL, University of Chicago Press, 1968

Saunders JB: The Transitions from Ancient Egyptian to Greek Medicine. Lawrence, KS, University of Kansas Press, 1963

Scarborough J: Roman Medicine. London, Thames and Hudson, 1969

Scotch N: Medical anthropology, in Biennial Review of Anthropology. Edited by Siegel BJ. Stanford, CA, Stanford University Press, 1963, pp 30–68

Shweder R, Bourne EJ: Does the concept of the person vary cross-culturally? in Cultural Conceptions of Mental Health and Therapy. Edited by Marsella AJ, White GM. Dordrecht, The Netherlands, D Reidel, 1982, pp 97–137

Stone DH: The Disabled State. Philadelphia, PA, Temple University Press, 1984

Temkin O: Scientific approach to disease, in Scientific Change: Historical Studies in the Intellectual, Social and Technical Conditions for Scientific Discovery and Technical Invention From Antiquity to the Present. Edited by Crombie AL. New York, Basic Books, 1963, pp 629–647

Temkin O: Galenism. New York, Cornell University Press, 1973

Ullman M: Islamic Surveys, Vol 2: Islamic Medicine. Edinburgh, Edinburgh University Press, 1978

Unschuld PU: Medicine in China: A History of Pharmaceutics. Berkeley, CA, University of California Press, 1983

Unschuld PU: Medicine in China: A History of Ideas. Berkeley, CA, University of California Press, 1985a

Unschuld PU: Medicine in China: Non-Ching, the Classic of Difficult Issues. Berkeley, CA, University of California Press, 1985b

Veith I: Hysteria: The History of a Disease. Chicago, IL, University of Chicago Press, 1965

Yanchi L: The Essential Book of Traditional Chinese Medicine. New York, Columbia University Press, 1988

Young A: Some implications of medical beliefs and practices for social anthropology. American Anthropologist 78:5–24, 1976

Chapter 10

Conclusion: Prospects for Research and Clinical Practice

Laurence J. Kirmayer, M.D., F.R.C.P.(C),
James M. Robbins, Ph.D.

I n this concluding chapter we explore some implications of the
work presented in this volume for current research and clinical
practice with somatizing patients. We also take this opportunity to
emphasize the importance of a number of topics that because of space
and organizational limitations could not be addressed or could only
be touched on by the contributors. We first address research issues
and then integrate research and clinical knowledge to offer guidelines
for treatment and social policy.

RESEARCH ISSUES

The fundamental issues raised by current work on somatization
include 1) the validity of dimensional versus categorical models of
psychiatric distress; 2) the utility of illness behavior versus
psychopathological models; 3) the limitations of self-report measures;
4) the role of emotional disturbance and expression; 5) the importance of a developmental, familial, and interpersonal perspective; 6)
the role of clinicians and the health care system; and, finally, 7) the
overarching social and cultural factors that shape the problem of
somatization.

Dimensional Versus Categorical Models

The "neo-Kraepelinian" approach of contemporary psychiatric nosology involves a search for discrete disorders characterized by distinctive
patterns of symptomatology. Modern psychiatry has been criticized
for its increasing emphasis on identification of discrete categories at
the expense of attention to processes common to seemingly disparate
syndromes (Kendell 1989; Mirowsky and Ross 1989). Categorical
thinking in psychiatry follows from the need to make binary decisions
in many aspects of clinical medicine. It is the physician's responsibility
to decide to treat or not to treat, to start or not to start a drug, and

201

to discharge or not to discharge a patient from the hospital (Klerman 1989). The emphasis on discrete diagnoses places psychiatry firmly within the larger tradition of biomedicine.

The current trend in psychiatric epidemiology toward interpreting continuous dimensions of human behavior as discontinuous disorders can also be traced to dissatisfaction with unitary concepts of mental illness and the assumption that different latent variables are responsible for different manifestations of mental disorder (Klerman 1989). Some justification for a categorical view of somatization comes from family studies suggesting a heritable component (Cloninger et al. 1984). Yet, the definitions of other somatoform disorders seem to identify symptoms or attributes rather than discrete entities.

It remains to be determined whether somatization is a continuous process, a process of discontinuous components, a composite of discrete functional somatic syndromes, or a distinct construct understandable only as an entity greater than the sum of its parts. To resolve these issues, researchers interested in somatization need to avoid arbitrary diagnostic cut points on continuous measures of somatization like the Diagnostic Interview Schedule (DIS) Somatic Symptom Index (SSI) or scores on a psychometric index of hypochondriasis. While it is often of value to know whether all criteria are met for a diagnosis, much information is lost when a continuous attribute is studied as either all present or all absent. Discontinuities in the number and pattern of unexplained medical symptoms or levels of hypochondriacal worry can be studied with newer statistical techniques, including latent variable analytic modeling (Grayson 1987; Grove et al. 1987; Swartz et al. 1986), Receiver Operating Curves (Smith and Brown 1990; Weinstein et al. 1989; Wilkinson and Markus 1989), and validation with external illness behavior criteria (Barsky et al. 1986; Escobar et al. 1987).

Illness Behavior Versus Psychopathological Models

Somatization can be viewed as a result of psychological disturbance or as the outcome of socially and culturally regulated patterns of illness behavior. Many plausible pathological models have been proposed. In Chapter 2, Pennebaker and Watson reviewed evidence for the constitutional predisposition of negative affectivity. This trait is associated with the tendency to experience and report all forms of distress. Along with Simon (Chapter 3), they summarized studies on individual differences in sensory-perceptual processes that may lead to an "amplifying somatic style" (Barsky and Klerman 1983). Characterological problems may also predispose individuals to somatic distress. A narcissistic investment in the body and its wholeness and perfect functioning may lead individuals to experience even minor physiological disruptions as devastating (Diamond 1987; Rodin 1984). On the other hand, somatization may serve defensive functions: some people may so fear psychological illness that they fixate on the somatic aspects of their suffering to avoid any confrontation with their own emotional conflict.

In contrast to these psychopathological models of somatization, the illness behavior perspective situates somatic distress within the social-psychological processes that govern all responses to potential illness (Mechanic 1983). Dispositions to attend to the body, to label sensations as symptoms, and to attribute these symptoms to disease or nondisease causes are thought to affect the outcome of all illness episodes (Angel and Thoits 1987; Kirmayer 1986; Robbins and Kirmayer 1986). These processes are identical to those that, when taken to an extreme, constitute an amplifying somatic style. Yet, the processes underlying different patterns of illness behavior need not in themselves be psychopathological.

Where illness behavior has been incorporated into psychiatric theory, it has often been translated from a normal process to a pathological condition (Pilowsky 1969). While the term has sometimes been used interchangeably with the sociological concept of "sick role," and has influenced the classification of disorders presenting with functional somatic symptoms, in psychiatry, illness behavior is often understood as "inappropriate" or "abnormal" illness behavior, meaning a pathological mode of responding to one's own state of health (Pilowsky 1990). This emphasis on pathology prejudges the significance of variations in illness behavior whose clinical implications are poorly understood (Mayou 1989).

It is likely that the most powerful explanatory model of somatization will combine the perspectives of psychopathology and illness behavior. Negative affectivity, for example, is thought to increase the perception of symptoms by causing one to be more self-focused and to anticipate negative events (Watson and Pennebaker 1989). Similarly, cognitive aspects of mood disorders may contribute directly to somatic preoccupation and symptom amplification. Anxiety, characterized by a sense of threat, vulnerability, and future-oriented catastrophizing, and depression with its pessimism and preoccupation with death, may lead to hypochondriacal worry and ruminations about sickness. Further, illness behavior may potentiate or mediate the stress-illness relationship (Stone and Neale 1981; Wickramasekera 1989). Interactive models that include measures of psychopathology, illness behavior, and the stress process may uncover hitherto obscured relationships with somatization.

The Limitations of Self-Report Measures

A methodological limitation of current models of somatization is that they almost exclusively employ self-report measures for both dependent and independent variables. In common with most cognitive social psychology, studies of somatization have relied on paper-and-pencil self-report measures because these are easy to apply. The meaning of these results is, however, more difficult to conceptualize (Kagan 1989). In defining somatization as high scores on somatic symptom self-reports or illness worry, investigators do not tap the patient's actual illness behavior. Recall of symptoms is influenced by context and demand characteristics that may lead subjects to under- or overestimate their actual levels. Existing measures cannot distinguish between the patient's actual experience and his or her conscious attempts to exaggerate distress or to dissimulate (Mendelson 1987).

It might be claimed, for example, that many hypochondriacal patients are unaware that they are hypochondriacal. However, because the hallmark of hypochondriasis is preoccupation and worry about disease, it is precisely because individuals' conscious awareness is often filled and focused on the possibility of disease that they are labeled hypochondriacal. Consequently, they are well able to report these concerns. Further, there is evidence that individuals who score persistently high on self-consciousness measures are more accurate in their self-assessments of emotional states and personality traits (Fenigstein et al. 1975). This finding suggests that self-reports of hypochondriacal individuals who are often self-focused are more likely to be accurate.

When self-report measures are used in an attempt to identify intervening variables that mediate the translation of sensations into distress, questions may make an implicit assumption that subjects have some awareness of these intervening processes. For example, subjects who are asked if they are very sensitive to pain or other sensations (e.g., "I can't stand pain as well as most people." "Sudden loud noises really disturb me.") (Barsky et al. 1988b) or those who are more sensitive than others, must make a comparative judgment vis-à-vis their standard of how others act. Such self-descriptions are often unreliable and are usually based not on introspection of a mediating process but on observation of one's own and others' behavior (Nisbett and Wilson 1977). As such these descriptions are measures of outcomes rather than mediating processes and may help little in characterizing the underlying mechanisms of symptom amplification.

The limitations of self-reports can be partly circumvented through the use of multiple measures to triangulate underlying constructs and develop a nomological network of interrelated latent constructs. This approach will lead to theoretical concepts that may be distant from the vocabulary of self-reports. For example, Kagan (1989) notes that the concept of negative affectivity is based entirely on self-reports. The underlying processes may be less accessible to self-report (e.g., early temperamental differences, autonomic instability, a strong physiological response to novelty, slow habituation or extinction of conditioned emotional response. These factors can be identified only with a broad range of measures including physiological and behavioral ones (e.g., James et al. 1989). As the processes leading to somatization are delineated, it will become possible to refine our definition and measures to rely less exclusively on self-report.

The Role of Affect

The relationship between affect and somatic distress is complex. Negative affective states or dysphoric moods are associated with increased levels of symptom reporting (Costa and McCrae 1980, 1985) and negative appraisals of one's own current health (Croyle and Uretsky 1987). In a study of the influence of daily variations in mood and fatigue in patients with lower-back pain, Feuerstein et al. (1987) found that anxiety and fatigue independently increased the level of pain experienced concurrently. No mood change was predictive of the onset of pain, but fatigue was elevated 24 hours after a pain episode. Thus, while dysphoric mood alone cannot account for many functional somatic symptoms, emotional distress and somatic distress form a positive feedback loop in which each form of suffering can intensify and perpetuate the other. This finding fits the observation that many patients with functional somatization also report high levels of anxious or depressed mood. Teasing apart the precise mediation of this vicious circle, which includes physiological, cognitive, and interpersonal processes, may lead to more effective clinical interventions.

Several lines of research converge on the notion that the inhibition or suppression of emotional expression can lead to prolonged states of physiological arousal and somatic distress (Beutler et al. 1986; Malatesta et al. 1987; Pennebaker and Beall 1986). We do not know if emotional expression in itself confers health benefits. Expression of strong emotion under conditions that allow optimal "cognitive distance" (or in the context of a protective relationship) may allow more rapid resolution of emotional arousal (Scheff 1984). Open acknowledgment of emotional distress may elicit support from intimate relationships or promote the identification and resolution of specific interpersonal conflicts. It is unclear whether the effects of suppression differ cross-culturally when the code for emotional expression varies (Kirmayer 1989). For example, where there are strong social prohibitions against the expression of specific emotions (e.g., anger, fear), two outcomes are possible: somatic distress may be more common or the expression of strong emotion may not confer health benefits because it is likely to be met with disapproval and rejection.

Clinical observations suggest that some patients with functional or psychologically aggravated somatic disorders have difficulty recounting their emotional experience and fantasy life. This suggestion has been interpreted as evidence of *alexithymia*—a deficit in the individual's capacity for verbal or symbolic elaboration and expression of emotion, conflict, and fantasy (Taylor 1984). It is unclear to what extent alexithymia is a stable personality trait or communicational style and whether it is a cause or consequence of somatic distress (Lesser and Lesser 1983). In many cases, patients are labeled alexithymic simply because their somatic preoccupation does not fit with the psychological orientation of the mental health practitioners they visit (Kirmayer 1987). With the development of improved measures (Bagby et al. 1988; Taylor and Bagby 1988), it may be possible to study the determinants of alexithymia and its role (if any) in somatization.

The Family-Developmental Perspective

While the individualistic perspective of Western psychiatry and psychology focuses on constitutional and personality factors in somatization, it is likely that many somatizing individuals are distinctive not for their own psychological traits but by virtue of the social context that shapes their illness behavior. For example, many psychologically minded individuals must adopt a somatic idiom of distress to have their suffering acknowledged by a spouse or significant other. Bodily expressions of distress may be less threatening to others than direct expressions of dissatisfaction with relationships. In these circumstances, somatization must be understood as a response to social predicaments rather than as an intrinsic property of the individual.

Even ostensible personality differences can be traced back to interpersonal processes in development. Early temperamental differences may predispose children to recurrent anxiety or persistent physiological arousal in situations where others remain calm. Parents who react to a child's somatic symptoms of anxiety by frequent visits to the doctor are likely to reinforce hypochondriacal preoccupations. At the same time, parental failure to identify and label specific emotions may leave the child unable to differentiate emotions from each other and from bodily distress of pathological significance. Thus, the components of the adult personality trait of negative affectivity may arise from simpler temperamental differences that are elaborated through family interaction to include features of excessive self-consciousness, poor self-image, and a sense of vulnerability to illness. The spectrum of traits found in an adult with a chronic hypochondriacal somatization disorder (Kellner's "developmental hypochondriasis"—see Chapter 8) may be the outcome of specific family processes interacting with the temperamental substrate of negative affectivity. Similarly, the phenomenon of alexithymia may be the outcome of family experiences where talk about emotions and conflict is prohibited or dismissed.

Wilkinson (1988) describes how differences in the family response to childhood illness episodes or "Monday morning stomachaches" may shape subsequent illness behavior. While clinical observations suggest that family dysfunction plays an important role in exacerbating somatic distress (Looff 1970; Minuchin et al. 1975; Wilkinson 1988), this effect appears to be nonspecific. The few empirical studies done have tended not to confirm specific relationships between family dysfunction and somatization (Walker et al. 1988). Unfortunately, existing measures of family functioning are often psychometrically unsatisfactory or do not tap dimensions of illness behavior and the communication of distress likely to be important in somatization. With modifications to measure emotional nonexpression or suppression, the work on expressed emotion and affective style (Leff and Vaughn 1985) might be profitably adapted to the study of families with somatizing members.

Somatization and the Health Care System

Studies of symptom variation must consider not just patients' experiences but practitioners' responses and the structure of the health care system as well. The form of patients' clinical presentation and subsequent illness experience is often a reflection of practitioner behavior that sanctions or ignores various forms of difficulty. Wickramasekera (1989) speaks of the conspiracy between doctor, patient, and insurer to resist psychosocial explanations for somatic disorders. For patients, a medical diagnosis avoids the stigma associated with mental illness. Medical diagnoses are reimbursed more readily than psychiatric ones. Physicians' fear of having "missed something," their lack of interest and training in assessing psychosocial aspects of distress, and the absence of well-validated psychosocial models of disease—all these support the practitioner's tendency to order extensive diagnostic tests, specialist consultations, and dubious treatments for patients with biomedically unexplained symptoms. Insurance companies, influenced in policy decisions by physicians and confused over the proliferation of mental health service providers who now apply for reimbursement rights, may find it simpler to encourage medical as opposed to psychosocial diagnoses.

Powerful social, legal, and financial aspects of the health care system act to reinforce a somatized communication of distress. There is evidence, however, that simple instructions to physicians may influence the health care demands of somatizing patients. Smith et al. (1986) conducted a randomized trial of psychiatric consultation in somatization disorder. They demonstrated that letters sent to physicians identifying and describing the characteristics of patients with somatization disorder, recommending regularly scheduled appointments for such patients, and cautioning against inappropriate assessments and hospitalizations, reduced the per capita expenditures on patients with somatization disorder by 53%. Interestingly, the expenditures for a substantial proportion of control patients—who were identified by their physicians as having recurrent somatic complaints but whose physicians did not receive the consultation letter—increased over the study period. This suggests that primary care physicians are capable of both reducing the morbidity of somatization and, perhaps by becoming more sensitive to the special cases, increasing it.

Somatizers often find their interactions with physicians frustrating, believing that they receive neither clear diagnosis nor effective treatment. As a result, alternative medicine may be particularly attractive to them. Of 395 patients attending a gastroenterology clinic studied by Verhoef et al. (1990), 33% of those with functional complaints had sought alternative medical care compared with only 7% of those with organic disease. The continued search for medical validation of subjective distress may lead somatizers to "doctor shop" beyond the conventional health care system.

Sociocultural Factors

Sociological studies have contributed greatly to our understanding of health and illness. Yet much remains to be learned of the social basis of somatization. Socioeconomic status has been identified as a factor in access to health care, exposure to health knowledge, and learned vocabularies of distress (Becker and Maiman 1983). Researchers have repeatedly found an inverse relationship between some forms of somatization and socioeconomic class, but we have few studies of how this relationship is mediated. Gender has been studied in the context of biological risk factors, healthy life-styles, and longevity (Verbrugge

1985), yet suggestions that women may be more sensitive to bodily sensations, willing to label symptoms as illness, and ready to take therapeutic action have not been systematically tested in somatization research. Sociologists have examined the role of social networks in helping sufferers interpret the meaning of symptoms, validate their distress, and obtain medical help (House et al. 1988), but here again the role of social support in somatization has not been adequately addressed. Theories of somatization are informed by the sociological concepts of sick role, illness behavior, and medicalization, yet a detailed analysis of the social and family worlds of somatizers is conspicuously absent from much current work on these conditions.

It has been repeatedly noted that, worldwide, somatization is a common—perhaps the most common—mode of expression of distress (Kirmayer 1984; Kleinman 1977). The anthropological study of somatization views it as one possible mode of expression of distress among many (Nichter 1981). Somatic distress commands attention, for it may reflect serious affliction that interferes with basic social roles and threatens life. Illness thus becomes a means of accumulating or consolidating power in social relationships, particularly for those whose other avenues to power are blocked. Thus, people trapped in difficult relationships or social circumstances and allowed little opportunity for direct criticism or protest may utilize somatic distress as a means of obtaining legitimate concern and concessions from local power structures as well as from larger social institutions (Kleinman 1986).

At the same time, the body provides natural symbols for social relationships and other salient aspects of culture (Kleinman 1986, 1988; O'Neill 1985; Scheper-Hughes and Lock 1987; Turner 1984). Somatic distress can then articulate quite specific social, moral, or religious concerns. Somatic symptoms have a symbolic meaning at social as well as psychological levels. Even when individuals are initially unaware of the symbolic meaning of their symptoms, they may be shaped by and may participate in social symbolic interaction or discourse.

This perspective may be helpful in understanding the cross-cultural differences found in epidemiologic studies. Cultural variations in illness models influence the experience and reporting of somatic symptoms (Kleinman 1980). For example, as reviewed in Chapter 4 of this volume, Rubio-Stipec and colleagues (1989) found different factor structures for responses to the DIS in Puerto Rico and at the United States National Institute of Mental Health Epidemiologic Catchment Area (ECA) sites. A prominent somatic factor was found in Puerto Rico that combined two of the clusters of symptoms previously identified by Swartz et al. (1986) using different statistical methods: one polysymptomatic cluster similar to somatization disorder and a second cluster consisting mainly of cardiorespiratory symptoms. This organization of symptoms may reflect the symptomatology of *nervios*, an indigenous illness category that links social stressors and traumatic events with a wide variety of anxiety symptoms and generalized somatic distress (Guarnaccia et al. 1989). The somatic referencing of social concerns and emotional distress is thus a basic cultural idiom of distress and joins together a broad range of somatic symptoms in a culturally coherent category. Such cultural models of illness can influence the perception of bodily sensations, leading individuals to label specific sensations as symptoms worthy of medical attention and to search for other symptoms that are expected to accompany them (Angel and Thoits 1987). Such cultural concepts of psychosomatic or sociosomatic relationships can then give rise to the interrelationships between symptoms observed at the epidemiologic level (Kirmayer 1984, 1989). The illness cognition approach we described in Chapter 6 offers a means of teasing apart some of the processes by which individuals come to display culturally distinctive modes of illness experience and behavior.

CLINICAL ISSUES

In the sections that follow, we outline some key clinical issues in the assessment and treatment of somatizing patients. Of necessity, these ideas go beyond what has been demonstrated by research—in part because of the perennial lack of methodologically sound outcome studies, but also because the clinical approach to somatizing patients, while grounded in scientific explanations of pathophysiology, psychology, and sociology, must also draw on the personal and cultural models that give the experience of illness meaning and coherence. The issues we consider include 1) the epistemological basis of the diagnosis of somatization; 2) somatic idioms of distress and the psychological mindedness of somatizing patients; 3) psychotherapeutic techniques derived from cognitive-behavioral psychodynamic and family systems perspectives; 4) the social management of the somatizing patient; 5) the place of narcissism and the therapeutic approach of self-psychology; 6) family therapy and systemic interventions; 7) the clinical and social policy aspects of the management of the somatizing patient in the health care, disability, and compensation systems; and, finally, 8) the cultural context of somatization as a sociomoral problem.

Clinical Epistemology of Functional Somatic Symptoms

Clinical diagnosis occurs in a context that does not allow many of the controls and experimental maneuvers basic to scientific investigation. As a result, there is often a much higher degree of ambiguity or uncertainty about the significance of signs and symptoms in individual patients than biomedical theory and the prototypical descriptions of diseases would suggest. The study of the limits of what is potentially knowable in the medical context might be termed *clinical epistemology*.

In practice, the term functional is often applied to symptoms that are simply medically unexplained. The DIS, for example, systematically inquires into whether the subject has received a medical diagnosis for each troubling somatic symptom. If the doctor had no explanation or the one reported by the patient is not plausible (according to current pathophysiological theory), then the symptom is scored as evidence of somatization. These symptoms would be more properly labeled idiopathic (i.e., of unknown origin) rather than functional.

There is never an absolute end to the process of ruling out organic disease; new technologies and advancing theory continue to offer patient and physician the option of ever more esoteric tests. Clinically, the decision that a symptom is unexplained then depends on a negotiated agreement between patient and physician to stop investigating and accept the state of uncertainty. This acceptance of uncertainty in turn reflects their willingness and ability to continue investigating; their acceptance of plausible or marginal explanations or tolerance of ambiguity and lack of closure; their ability to resolve or deny the worry and uncertainty introduced by uncomfortable and possibly disabling symptoms; and their ability to control symptoms (despite a lack of diagnosis). Forces at work in the social contexts of both physician and patient tend to work against any acceptance of "not knowing" as a satisfactory end point in medical investigation. Patients are left anxious and uncertain; physicians must confront limits to their expertise and competence and face the difficult task of working with worried or querulous patients. Institutions may demand that symptoms be labeled and categorized in ways that allow standard treatment and reimbursement, and define liability and disability. The strong tendency to label idiopathic symptoms "functional," and to further attribute functional symptoms to specific psychological causes, can be understood in the context of this profound discomfort with not knowing.

While labeling a symptom functional ought to carry no strict implication about its relationship to psychosocial factors, in fact, it is often one step toward attributing the symptom to psychological causes. Clinically, the clear demonstration that a symptom is psychogenic is rarely possible. Several types of evidence are commonly used to establish a connection between a symptom and a psychosocial cause or context, but each has serious limitations:

1. *Contiguity.* Symptom onset is preceded by a clear-cut psychosocial stressor. Occasionally, symptoms will come and go in strict association with a salient psychological event or state, and this will allow a degree of confidence that the psychological factor is contributory. Far more commonly, potential psychosocial contributors are identified, but it cannot be precisely ascertained whether they antedated the symptom or arose in conjunction with it. The recollection of recent life events may be biased by the tendency to search for explanations and reassess the negativity of events once a symptom has developed. Further, individuals who are symptomatic may have their coping impaired and so be more vulnerable to untoward life events.

2. *Intensity.* Antecedent or ongoing stressors of sufficient intensity exist to account for the symptomatology. It is not only the presence but the severity of stressors that makes them plausible causes for somatic distress. A severe loss or change in social status is viewed as sufficient to account for comparably severe somatic distress. The problem here is that there are few reliable measures of the severity of a stressor that depends on the personal meaning of events and the individual's idiosyncratic judgment of his or her ability to cope adequately with the challenge. Estimates of the intensity of social stress are thus confounded with the symptomatic distress that they are intended to explain.

3. *Personality.* When no serious life events can be identified, the patient's personality or psychological state may be invoked as a cause of excessive vulnerability to ordinary levels of stress or as a source of symptom-generating conflict in its own right. Personality difficulties, by definition, have usually long anteceded the symptom and so cannot easily explain its occurrence at a particular point in time. Acute psychological distress (and personality changes) may just as well be a concomitant effect of the same processes that give rise to somatic distress, or a consequence of persistent somatic symptoms.

4. *Causal theories.* The search for contiguity, intensity, and personality dimensions that could account for the link between functional symptoms and psychosocial factors is guided by existing theories of causal processes. Where such a theory is accepted, any factors

that correlate with its explanatory constructs will be included as additional evidence for the psychogenic nature of symptoms. For example, the assumption that attention and reward can reinforce symptoms leads to the tendency to identify "secondary gain" not only as evidence of factors that cause symptoms to persist but also as evidence that symptoms were psychological in the first instance.

5. *Symbolic meaning.* Symptoms are communicative acts, whether intended as such or not, and can be decoded with reference to personal, contextual, and cultural notions of meaningfulness (Kirmayer 1987; Kleinman 1988). When socially significant meaning can be ascribed to symptoms, this can be used to classify them as predominantly social actions and hence to impute psychosocial causation.

As can be seen from these examples, the identification of psychological factors that accompany or even exacerbate a symptom is often incorrectly adduced as evidence that the symptom itself is psychogenic. The covariation of symptom severity with psychological distress establishes a link but does not distinguish functional symptoms from those with obvious organic causes: patients with organic pain also experience worsening in conjunction with stressful events and amelioration with the improvement of their emotional and social condition.

There are several points worth noting about these epistemological considerations. The attribution of a somatic symptom to a stressor depends in large part on available theories of psychosomatic causation. Clinicians who have more global theories of psychosomatic causation may be more willing to connect patients' symptoms to psychosocial factors. Advancing knowledge of psychophysiological processes may make some forms of stress-symptom connection seem plausible while others become more far-fetched. Overarching these theoretical issues are the patient and clinician's general attitudes of acceptance or willingness to consider psychological or emotional factors in distress. When the attitude toward these factors is negative (because of unfamiliarity, skepticism, or defensiveness), the attribution will be made less often. Patients whom we have other reasons for not liking, or who irritate or frustrate clinicians, will be more likely to receive a "functional" or psychogenic diagnosis.

In most cases ambiguity remains. Thus, the clinician's insistence on a somatizing interpretation must be understood with regard to the ultimate clinical (or personal or institutional) goals. The clinical goal ought to be to help the patient. Hence, we should ask whether the labeling of a problem as somatization leads to some corrective action that will benefit the patient. Often, other conflicting goals intervene: the personal desire of the clinician to maintain his authority and competence in the eyes of patients and colleagues and institutional goals to assign definite diagnoses and delimit professional responsibility for intractable problems. These goals, while not in themselves base, may conflict with the delivery of optimal care to the individual patient.

Somatic Idioms of Distress and Psychological Mindedness

Psychologically oriented practitioners have found it difficult to form working alliances with somatically preoccupied patients and have assumed that somatization has a poor outcome. At the same time, many physicians have found functional symptoms difficult to diagnose and treat. Consequently, somatizing patients have tended to fall between the chairs of medical and psychiatric expertise. Recognizing that clinicians are confused or stumped by their problems, many somatizing patients engage in an earnest search for alternative forms of care that may be more comforting and helpful (Verhoef et al. 1990). By resorting to alternative modes of health care these patients may further undermine the legitimacy of their health concerns in the view of biomedical practitioners.

While many patients with medically unexplained somatic symptoms may be suffering from major depressions or other psychiatric disorders, they tend to attribute their distress to physical causes. This attribution seems natural in view of the somatic nature of their symptomatology. Whether the clinician can identify a treatable psychiatric disorder or not, the first need of these patients is to have the somatic reality of their suffering acknowledged. Too often, psychologically oriented practitioners discount somatic symptoms in favor of familiar forms of emotional distress. Somatizing patients are often depicted as not psychologically minded and therefore not amenable to conventional psychotherapy. The anthropological view of somatic symptoms as part of a local idiom of distress is a helpful corrective to this impatience with patients' preeminent concerns. The development of behavioral medicine techniques has also made it easier to approach somatizing patients through an explicit focus on their somatic distress (Garrick and Loewenstein 1989; Ford and Parker, Chapter 7, this volume). When the somatic nature of the illness is accepted, many patients are able to consider emotional and interpersonal dimensions as well and often introduce these dimensions themselves.

Patients who continue to completely reject psychosocial aspects of their distress fall into three broad categories: 1) those whose physical distress is so intense and pressing that it occludes awareness of other dimensions until its urgency is met; 2) those who have a continuing need for medical legitimation of the somatic nature of their illness usually because of the skepticism of some important other—for example, a family member, employer, compensation board, or insurance company; and 3) those who privately or unconsciously feel that their psychosocial problems are unmanageable or inescapable. Working with the first group calls for the application of effective means of symptom control to reduce the intensity and urgency of distress. Working with the second demands an assessment of the systemic factors maintaining the sick role, followed by family or social network interventions to change the meaning of the somatic distress. Working with the third group requires the development of a more supportive therapeutic relationship in which the patient can gradually become less fearful of his or her own thoughts and feelings and so admit more of them to consciousness. In each case, these strategies can proceed only if the bodily nature of the patients' suffering continues to be acknowledged and explored.

Therapeutic Strategies

A variety of cognitive-behavioral techniques devised for depression and anxiety are readily adapted to patients with somatization. Relaxation training allows patients to learn patterns of physiological response that reduce symptomatology and interfere with the emotional hyperarousal that may contribute to somatic distress (Poppen 1988). Stress-management techniques based on problem solving, cognitive restructuring, and enhancement of self-efficacy act nonspecifically to reduce somatic distress by decreasing the impact of stressful events and improving coping with symptoms (Litt and Baker 1987; Meichenbaum 1985). Biofeedback offers a way to alter physiological function that seems particularly appropriate for functional syndromes (Schwartz et al. 1987). The explicit focus on physical sensations and the use of technical apparatus may also serve to ratify the patient's perception of his or her problem as physical even while he or she is learning new ways of coping.

Specific cognitive-behavioral techniques can target self- and body-consciousness, hypochondriacal worry and thoughts of illness vulnerability, and attributional style. One approach likely to benefit some patients with functional or hypochondriacal symptoms involves learning to reattribute common somatic symptoms to benign sources (Barsky et al. 1988a; Gask et al. 1989; Goldberg et al. 1989; Wessely et al. 1989).

There is evidence that hypochondriacal fears can be treated like

other phobias by exposure to the feared stimuli and response prevention (Warwick and Marks 1988). The success of this therapeutic
approach supports the idea that clinicians and family members may
inadvertently reinforce hypochondriasis by responding to the
patient's requests for reassurance. The challenge for the clinician is to
develop the sort of working alliance with the patient in which the
illness maintaining patterns of interaction can be interrupted. When
somatic symptoms appear to be maintained by social contingencies,
family and systemic interventions may be most effective (McDaniel et
al. 1989; Patterson and Spees 1988). Assertiveness training may enable individuals to obtain power in relationships without the use of
the sick role.

Cognitive psychotherapy emphasizes the individual's ability to
achieve control over distressing symptoms and circumstances. For
many somatizing patients this has immediate appeal. There are situations, however, where the effort to control these circumstances may
be problematic and give rise to symptoms through cycles of emotional
exacerbation (Kirmayer 1990). Strategic interventions may provide
rapid relief by interrupting the effortful striving that maintains
symptoms and somatic preoccupation. Training in self-hypnosis can
afford symptom control and also increase cognitive flexibility and
tolerance of "letting go" when appropriate (Crasilneck and Hall
1985; Golden et al. 1987; Spiegel 1988).

Patients who are unable to differentiate bodily sensations that
indicate disease from those that are benign or ordinary concomitants
of emotion can be taught to discriminate their emotions through
experiential therapies. For some patients, intolerance of physiological
and emotional arousal reflects more pervasive defects in self-image
and self-regulation. Insight-oriented and relational therapies may
allow patients to develop more stable self-cohesion and tolerance of
strong affect (Diamond 1987; Rodin 1984).

Social Management

Treatment of somatizers is often unsuccessful and unrewarding for
both the patient and the physician. Patients are motivated to seek help
for relief of distressing symptoms and for social validation of personal
suffering. Because symptoms are a subjective reality, sufferers must
rely on biomedical experts to validate claims of discomfort. When
somatizers visit the physician and do so repeatedly, the result is often
yet another test or yet another referral to a specialist. After these
avenues have been exhausted, the physician may eventually offer a
psychological explanation and prescribe psychotherapy, tranquilizers,
or stress reduction. Or worse, he or she may conclude that the patient

is malingering and that the symptoms are imaginary (Lennon et al. 1989).

Often the patient will respond to a psychological explanation or referral with skepticism or frustration, leaving the appointment frustrated or angry that the doctor cannot see how much the patient's body hurts. The patient is unable to understand how unconscious conflict, family dysfunction, habitual behavior patterns, or perturbed neurotransmitters can account for his or her suffering. If the physician is successful in getting somatizers to try psychotherapy, they are likely to think the ideas silly and not worthy of serious attention. If they say so, the therapist is likely to conclude that the patient is psychologically defended and resistant to psychological insight. When they stop coming to therapy, they are classified as treatment failures, dropouts, or "noncompliers," as though it is entirely their own fault and not a failure of clinical care.

To understand why psychological explanations are anathema to somatizers, we should consider the possibility, for example, that there is resistance to the stigma of a diagnosis that suggests mental illness; that the pain or distress of somatizers is experienced as a bodily, not a mental, problem; or that somatizers are simply correct and psychological explanations are inappropriate. We must seriously consider whether a patient is simply telling us the truth when he or she says, "There are no psychological causes for my symptoms; I am not inhibited in my emotional expression; I am not really depressed, even when I look deep into my psyche like you insist that I must."

What alternatives can we offer somatizing patients who are not amenable to conventional psychiatric care? From research on somatization, we can suggest that different forms of what we call somatization are best managed by different approaches. First, it is known that some somatizers are psychiatrically disturbed at the time that they present to the doctor. Many somatizing presenters are severely dysphoric and will frankly acknowledge psychosocial stressors when interviewed by a skilled clinician. These patients are likely to accept psychiatric referral when evaluation and treatment follow the guidelines discussed above. There is evidence, however, that some somatizers are not intensely dysphoric and make no connection between their physical complaints and psychological worries (Goldberg and Bridges 1988). Hence, they may be poor candidates for psychiatric referral. These patients may be most appropriately managed by primary care providers who are adequately trained to provide thorough psychiatric evaluation in a general medical setting. These clinicians are best positioned to integrate both medical and psychological care and to reevaluate changes in symptomatology that may herald new disease.

Other somatizers have a history of multiple unexplained somatic symptoms but are without a psychiatric disorder. Of those, many have co-occurring hypochondriacal worry that seems to be associated with heightened body consciousness and self-focus, pathological symptom attributions, and help seeking. A different group has a history of functional symptoms without extraordinary hypochondriasis. They are not conscious of amplified body perception but will likely continue to present with many complaints. In both of these cases, the physician should first accept their distress as physically, and not psychologically, based. Unqualified understanding and acceptance alone may support the somatizer's self-esteem such that he or she will be better able to cope with ongoing symptoms (Pearlin et al. 1981).

Among patients with a long history of functional symptoms and coexisting hypochondriacal worry, the physician should consider offering specific reassurance, complete and unambiguous medical information, and systematic education in the normal psychology of bodily symptoms, along with stress reduction techniques to minimize disability and maximize functioning. These patients should be told that they have physical symptoms of which we do not know the cause, but that the symptoms will almost certainly not shorten their lives and that there are ways to help them live with these symptoms. In addition, referral should be considered. The ideal referral would be to a specific *illness adaptation program*. In such a program, patients would 1) learn more about their condition—most importantly, that it is not life threatening; 2) learn to accept that medicine has limitations and that one cannot expect there to be a cure for everything (Barsky 1988); 3) learn that others suffer from similar complaints but are not particularly disabled by them; and 4) learn skills to cope with symptoms. The program would also state explicitly that even if symptoms cannot be alleviated, the incapacitating worry that substantially increases illness behavior can be (Robbins et al. 1990). If appropriate, patients might be taught skills to dampen bodily sensitivity, refocus their preoccupation with illness, and normalize new bodily sensations. Barsky and colleagues (1988a) are developing a program along these lines.

Somatizers without hypochondriacal beliefs may have less tolerance for educational programs such as described above, since they may be less emotionally invested in their somatic symptoms. In these cases, it is the treating physicians, not the patient, who should perhaps be "managed." Smith et al. (1986) have illustrated exactly how getting physicians to adhere to a structured protocol can influence the health care utilization of patients with somatization disorder. Following this model, physicians should be trained to schedule regular visits with somatizing patients. In this way future visits will not be contingent on generation of new symptoms. Visits should focus on symptomatic relief and reassurance, not on additional diagnostic procedures. Physicians should also be taught that somatizing patients are at high risk for inappropriate hospitalizations.

Somatization as a Sociomoral Problem

The concept of somatization is rooted in the dualistic metaphysics of Western medicine: it implies that distress, which is fundamentally psychological or social in origin and nature, is transformed into or expressed as somatic distress. For many non-Western cultures, as Fabrega (see Chapter 9, this volume) illustrates, emotions, thought, and social relations are inseparable from bodily sensations. Hence, the somatic experience and expression of distress in response to personal or familial problems do not constitute a puzzling fact to be explained by psychopathology. Instead, they are an inevitable consequence of the interrelatedness of mind and body.

In Western psychiatry, where an underlying dualism persists, there is an inescapable moral dimension to psychosomatic diagnosis. Illness is either attributed to impersonal causes and viewed as an accident that befalls the patient as victim, or is viewed as psychologically caused and mediated and, hence, potentially under the person's voluntary control. When control is imputed, whether actual or potential, the patient may be viewed as causing his or her own illness. Even when psychologically sophisticated clinicians attempt to adopt a holistic perspective, they must contend with pervasive notions of dualism that are implicit in the cultural concept of the person (Kirmayer 1988). Patients and their families may insist on knowing whether the problem is physical or psychological, real or imaginary, accidental or self-imposed.

It is unfortunate that useful ideas about psychosocial contributors to distress become caught up in issues of the "reality" of distress. In part, it is because functional disorders have no definite publicly verifiable correlate by which their presence and progress can be marked that we give them a lesser or defective ontological status. It is also because we presume that functional symptoms are associated with psychological factors such as personality, volition, and life-style that we accord them a different moral status from organic disease. The morally pejorative connotations of psychosomatic diagnosis present serious social problems for many patients with functional somatic disorders who feel that their problems are being treated as "not real" and due to their psychological disability or moral culpability. Physicians who adopt a hierarchical-systems view that acknowledges the reality of functional symptoms must still face the pervasive dualism of Western society that seeks to partition ill fortune into accident and intention and to ascribe personal causation, responsibility, and blame to problems of psychological origin (Kirmayer 1988). A comprehensive clinical perspective must contend with this dualism to educate patients, families, and society about the unified nature of disease and distress and the moral distinctions among causation, responsibility, and blame.

REFERENCES

Angel R, Thoits P: The impact of culture on the cognitive structure of illness. Cult Med Psychiatry 11:465–494, 1987

Bagby RM, Taylor GJ, Atkinson L: Alexithymia: a comparative study of three self-report measures. J Psychosom Res 32:107–116, 1988

Barsky AJ: The paradox of health. New Engl J Med 318:414–418, 1988

Barsky AJ, Klerman GL: Overview: hypochondriasis, bodily complaints, and somatic styles. Am J Psychiatry 140:273–283, 1983

Barsky AJ, Wyshak G, Klerman GL: Medical and psychiatric determinants of outpatient medical utilization. Med Care 24:548–560, 1986

Barsky AJ, Geringer E, Wool CA: A cognitive-educational treatment for hypochondriasis. Gen Hosp Psychiatry 10:322–327, 1988a

Barsky AJ, Goodson JD, Lane RS, et al: The amplification of somatic symptoms. Psychosom Med 50:510–519, 1988b

Becker MH, Maiman LA: Models of health-related behavior, in Handbook of Health, Health Care, and the Health Professions. Edited by Mechanic D. New York, Free Press, 1983, pp 539–568

Beutler LE, Oro'-Beutler ME, Daldrup R, et al: Inability to express intense affect: a common link between depression and pain? J Consult Clin Psychol 54:752–759, 1986

Cloninger CR, Sigvardsson S, von Knorring A-L, et al: An adoption study of somatoform disorders, II: Identification of two discrete somatoform disorders. Arch Gen Psychiatry 41:863–871, 1984

Costa PT Jr, McCrae RR: Somatic complaints in males as a function of age and neuroticism: a longitudinal analysis. J Behav Med 3:245–255, 1980

Costa PT Jr, McCrae RR: Hypochondriasis, neuroticism, and aging: when are somatic complaints unfounded? Am Psychol 40:19–28, 1985

Crasilneck HD, Hall JA: Clinical Hypnosis: Principles and Applications, Second Edition. New York, Grune & Stratton, 1985

Croyle RT, Uretsky MF: Effects of mood on self-appraisal of health status. Health Psychol 6:239–253, 1987

Diamond DB: Psychotherapeutic approaches to the treatment of panic attacks, hypochondriasis and agoraphobia. Br J Med Psychol 60:79–84, 1987

Escobar JI, Golding JM, Hough RL, et al: Somatization in the community: relationship to disability and use of services. Am J Public Health 77:837–840, 1987

Feuerstein M, Carter RL, Papciak AS: A prospective analysis of stress and fatigue in recurrent low back pain. Pain 31:333–344, 1987

Fenigstein A, Scheier MF, Buss AH: Public and private self-consciousness: assessment and theory. J Consult Clin Psychol 43:522–527, 1975

Garrick TR, Loewenstein RJ: Behavioral medicine in the general hospital. Psychosomatics 30:123–134, 1989

Gask L, Goldberg D, Porter R, et al: The treatment of somatization: evaluation of a teaching package with general practice trainees. J Psychosom Res 33:697–703, 1989

Goldberg DP, Bridges K: Somatic presentations of psychiatric illness in primary care setting. J Psychosom Res 32:137–144, 1988

Goldberg D, Gask L, O'Dowd T: The treatment of somatization: teaching techniques of reattribution. J Psychosom Res 33:689–695, 1989

Golden WL, Dowd ET, Friedberg F: Hypnotherapy: A Modern Approach. New York, Pergamon, 1987

Grayson D: Can categorical and dimensional views of psychiatric illness be distinguished? Br J Psychiatry 151:355–361, 1987

Grove WM, Andreasen NC, Young M, et al: Isolation and characterization of a nuclear depressive syndrome. Psychol Med 17:471–484, 1987

Guarnaccia PJ, Rubio SM, Canino G: Ataques de nervios in the Puerto Rican diagnostic interview schedule: the impact of cultural categories on psychiatric epidemiology. Cult Med Psychiatry 13:275–295, 1989

House JS, Landis KR, Umberson D: Social relationships and health. Science 241:540–545, 1988

James L, Gordon E, Kraiuhin C, et al: Selective attention and auditory event-related potentials in somatization disorder. Compr Psychiatry 30:84–89, 1989

Kagan J: Unstable Ideas: Temperament, Cognition and Self. Cambridge, MA, Harvard University Press, 1989

Kendell RE: Clinical validity. Psychol Med 19:45–55, 1989

Kirmayer LJ: Culture, affect and somatization. Transcultural Psychiatric Research Review 21:159–188, 237–262, 1984

Kirmayer LJ: Somatization and the social construction of illness experience, in Illness Behavior: A Multidisciplinary Perspective. Edited by McHugh S, Vallis TM. New York, Plenum, 1986, pp 111–133

Kirmayer LJ: Languages of suffering and healing: alexithymia as a social and cultural process. Transcultural Psychiatric Research Review 24:119–136, 1987

Kirmayer LJ: Mind and body as metaphors: hidden values in biomedicine, in Biomedicine Examined. Edited by Lock M, Gordon D. Dordrecht, The Netherlands, Kluwer, 1988, pp 57–92

Kirmayer LJ: Cultural variations in the response to psychiatric disorders and emotional distress. Soc Sci Med 29:327–339, 1989

Kirmayer LJ: Resistance, reactance and reluctance to change: a cognitive attributional approach to strategic interventions. Journal of Cognitive Psychotherapy 4:83–104, 1990

Kleinman A: Depression, somatization and the "new cross-cultural psychiatry." Soc Sci Med 11:3–10, 1977

Kleinman A: Patients and Healers in the Context of Culture. Berkeley, CA, University of California Press, 1980

Kleinman A: Social Origins of Distress and Disease. New Haven, CT, Yale University Press, 1986

Kleinman A: The Illness Narratives: Suffering, Healing and the Human Condition. New York, Harper & Row, 1988

Klerman G: Psychiatric diagnostic categories: issues in validity and measurement. J Health Soc Behav 30:26–32, 1989

Leff J, Vaughn C: Expressed Emotion in Families. New York, Guilford, 1985

Lennon MC, Link BG, Marbach JJ, et al: The stigma of chronic facial pain and its impact on social relationships. Social Problems 36:117–134, 1989

Lesser IM, Lesser BZ: Alexithymia: examining the development of a psychological concept. Am J Psychiatry 140:1305–1308, 1983

Litt MD, Baker LH: Cognitive-behavioral intervention for irritable bowel syndrome. J Clin Gastroenterol 9:208–211, 1987

Looff DH: Psychophysiologic and conversion reactions in children—selective incidence in verbal and nonverbal families. J Am Acad Child Psychiatry 9:318–331, 1970

Malatesta C, Jonas R, Izard CE: The relation between low facial expressivity during emotional arousal and somatic symptoms. Br J Med Psychol 60:169–180, 1987

Mayou R: Illness behavior and psychiatry. Gen Hosp Psychiatry 11:307–312, 1989

McDaniel SH, Campbell T, Seaburn D: Somatic fixation in patients and physicians: a biopsychosocial approach. Family Systems Medicine 7:5–16, 1989

Mechanic D: The experience and expression of distress: the study of illness behavior and medical utilization, in Handbook of Health, Health Care, and the Health Professions. Edited by Mechanic D. New York, Free Press, 1983, pp 591–607

Meichenbaum D: Stress Inoculation Training. New York, Pergamon, 1985

Mendelson G: Measurement of conscious symptom exaggeration by questionnaire: a clinical study. J Psychosom Res 31:703–712, 1987

Minuchin S, Baker L, Rosman BL, et al: A conceptual model of psychosomatic illness in children: family organization and family therapy. Arch Gen Psychiatry 32:1031–1038, 1975

Mirowsky J, Ross CE: Psychiatric diagnosis as reified measurement. J Health Soc Behav 30:11–25, 1989

Nichter M: Idioms of distress: alternatives in the expression of psychosocial distress: a case study from India. Cult Med Psychiatry 5:379–408, 1981

Nisbett RE, Wilson TD: Telling more than we can know: verbal reports on mental processes. Psychol Rev 84:231–259, 1977

O'Neill J: Five Bodies: The Human Shape of Modern Society. Ithaca, NY, Cornell University Press, 1985

Patterson JE, Spees DN: Considering the options: a multilevel systemic approach to helping somatizing patients. Family Systems Medicine 6:411–420, 1988

Pearlin LI, Lieberman MA, Menaghan EG, et al: The stress process. J Health Soc Behav 22:337–356, 1981

Pennebaker JW, Beall SK: Confronting a traumatic event: toward an understanding of inhibition and disease. J Abnorm Psychol 95:274–281, 1986

Pilowsky I: Abnormal illness behaviour. Br J Med Psychol 42:347–351, 1969

Pilowsky I: The concept of abnormal illness behavior. Psychosomatics 31:207–213, 1990

Poppen R: Behavioral Relaxation Training and Assessment. New York, Pergamon, 1988

Robbins JM, Kirmayer LJ: Illness cognition, symptom reporting and somatization in primary care, in Illness Behavior: A Multidisciplinary Model. Edited by McHugh S, Vallis TM. New York, Plenum, 1986, pp 283–302

Robbins JM, Kirmayer LJ, Kapusta MA: Illness worry and disability in fibromyalgia syndrome. Int J Psychiatry Med 20:49–63, 1990

Rodin G: Somatization and the self: psychotherapeutic issues. Am J Psychother 38:257–263, 1984

Rubio-Stipec M, Shrout P, Bird H, et al: Symptom scales of the Diagnostic Interview Schedule: factor results in Hispanic and Anglo samples. J Consult Clin Psychol 1:30–34, 1989

Scheff T: The taboo on coarse emotions, in Review of Personality and Social Psychology, Vol 5. Edited by Shaver P. Beverly Hills, CA, Sage, 1984, pp 146–169

Scheper-Hughes N, Lock M: The mindful body: a prolegomenon to future work in medical anthropology. Med Anthropol 1:6–41, 1987

Schwartz MS, et al: Biofeedback: A Practitioner's Guide. New York, Guilford, 1987

Smith GR Jr, Brown FW: Screening indexes in DSM-III-R somatization disorder. Gen Hosp Psychiatry 12:148–152, 1990

Smith GR, Monson RA, Ray G: Psychiatric consultation in somatization disorder. N Engl J Med 314:1407–1413, 1986

Spiegel D: Hypnosis, in American Psychiatric Press Textbook of Psychiatry. Edited by Talbott JA, Hales RE, Yudofsky SC. Washington, DC, American Psychiatric Press, 1988, pp 907–928

Stone AA, Neale JM: Hypochondriasis and tendency to adopt the sick role as moderators of the relationship between life-events and somatic symptomatology. Br J Med Psychol 54:75–81, 1981

Swartz M, Blazer D, Woodbury M, et al: Somatization disorder in a U.S. southern community: use of a new procedure for analysis of medical classification. Psychol Med 16:595–609, 1986

Taylor GJ: Alexithymia: concept, measurement, and implications for treatment. Am J Psychiatry 141:725–732, 1984

Taylor GJ, Bagby RM: Measurement of alexithymia: recommendations for clinical practice and future research. Psychiatr Clin North Am 11:351–366, 1988

Turner BS: The Body and Society. New York, Basil Blackwell, 1984

Verbrugge L: Gender and health: an update on hypotheses and evidence. J Health Soc Behav 26:157–177, 1985

Verhoef MJ, Sutherland LR, Brkich L: Use of alternative medicine by patients attending a gastroenterology clinic. Can Med Assoc J 142:121–125, 1990

Walker LS, McLaughlin FJ, Greene JW: Functional illness and family functioning: a comparison of health and somaticizing adolescents. Fam Process 27:317–320, 1988

Warwick HMC, Marks IM: Behavioural treatment of illness phobia and hypochondriasis: a pilot study of 17 cases. Br J Psychiatry 152:239–241, 1988

Watson D, Pennebaker JW: Health complaints, stress and distress: exploring the central role of negative affectivity. Psychol Rev 96:234–254, 1989

Weinstein MC, Berwick DM, Goldman PA, et al: A comparison of three psychiatric screening tests using Receiver Operating Characteristic (ROC) analysis. Med Care 27:593–607, 1989

Wessely S, David A, Butler S, et al: Management of chronic (post-viral) fatigue syndrome. J R Coll Gen Pract 39:26–29, 1989

Wickramasekera I: Enabling the somatizing patient to exit the somatic closet: a high-risk model. Psychotherapy 26:530–544, 1989

Wilkinson SR: The Child's World of Illness: The Development of Health and Illness Behaviour. Cambridge, UK, Cambridge University Press, 1988

Wilkinson G, Markus AC: Validation of a computerized assessment (PROQSY) of minor psychological morbidity by Relative Operating Characteristic analysis using a single GP's assessments as criterion measures. Psychol Med 19:225–231, 1989

Index

227